WELLNESS REFLECTION

New Journey Book & Journal

CONTENTS

WHAT'S BEHIND WEIGHT GAIN?

Y ou are fabulous, fun, and fierce. No matter the number on your scale or the size of your waistline, you are a vibrant and powerful woman.

You deserve health and vitality, regardless of your age.

Everywhere I look, though, women do not feel fierce or fabulous. Women today, especially as they get older, feel overweight, overwhelmed, and discouraged.

In fact, women over 40 are among the least satisfied, least healthy, and least happy people in America.

In America today, the way we think and talk about health and beauty makes us feel less-than, and therefore worthless.

In an age of chronic stress, competition, and unhealthy beauty standards, women of all ages (especially women over 40) are blocked from achieving their full potential. Because we are made to feel less-than-perfect, we are limited in our paths to achieving the fitness goals we so earnestly pursue.

I have seen so many women in my age group feeling unmotivated, unhappy, unsatisfied, and even depressed as they age. If any of those traits describes you, that can all change in a short period of time with just a little consistent effort!

Now, let's get started on your path to higher energy, feeling happier, and a having healthier lifestyle, inside and out.

We may sometimes feel a decline in vitality as we age, due to the imbalance of our wellness in mind, body, and spirit.

That can change. Here's how...

We are taught that we have the right to the *pursuit* of happiness, not happiness itself.

Western culture teaches that humans have the right to life, liberty, and the pursuit of happiness. For many of us, though, happiness is far from reach.

Today, happiness is tied to physical factors such as age, weight, income level, marital status, educational level, and other arbitrary measures of worth. No wonder we all struggle to feel like we measure up! There are simply too many ways to fall short.

Society further defines what happiness is. Instead of allowing us to find our own path to our own happiness, we are taught that we have to reach certain goals by certain ages, or we fail. We have to be a certain weight, a certain height, eat certain things, like certain things, and meet certain expectations or we are just not happy.

And why wouldn't everyone want to be happy?

Happiness, all too often, is just something we chase, not something we achieve. It's too steeped in unrealistic expectations of beauty, wealth, and status, most of which contradict each other.

As a result, we find ourselves overweight, overtaxed, and overwhelmed. Women over 40 are especially vulnerable, due to the stresses of caring for others and themselves through the trickiest part of life. Hormonal changes during this time create added stress and difficulty when it comes to exercising and dieting, leaving us exhausted and dissatisfied. Losing weight at this time can seem impossible, and no wonder. These challenges seem unsurmountable at times.

However, mid-life does not have to be the toughest part of life. Mid-life and beyond can be your best years.

My experience in fitness and health comes from years of healing. I'm a National Physique Committee (NPC) athlete, and, up until the writing of this book, have been competing for four years, always placing in the top five in my category. I also have with years of teaching dance and fitness. My love for fitness began when I experienced the Insanity program and further grew when I was exposed to the Shape Up America initiative, when I had the opportunity to work in my community. As a certified group fitness instructor, I encourage and motivate people to achieve and enjoy a healthy, fit lifestyle with lasting results. As a dancer, I combine my loves for movement and health to assist people like you to feel better in every possible way.

Although I never struggled with extra weight, I did have body satisfaction issues and I understand the root cause of the problem of putting on and being unable to get rid of extra weight. I know what it's like to be dissatisfied. I have felt the emotional pain of not liking my body, not feeling good enough, being stressed out, and not loving myself. Also, I have worked with hundreds of clients, helping them achieve their weight goals.

When I was younger, I trained as a ballet dancer. My body was great for dancing, but I didn't think I was attractive for anything else. Being a black girl and shaped like a rectangle felt like a problem, and as I grew into a young adult, I was highly self-conscious and believed everyone else looked better than me. Over the years I figured out how to change my shape: put on some muscle, create some curves, and get amazingly fit and healthy in the process. You can do the same.

This book will unpack a variety of factors behind body dissatisfaction and weight troubles for women over 40. If you are in this category (or are reading on behalf of someone in this category), you probably understand the difficulties of aging in Western society.

The trouble is that "happiness" is so poorly defined and so fleeting that most of us, sooner or later, find ourselves in deep waters. In particular, women over 40 in the United States are statistically the least satisfied with their lives, and no wonder. For many reasons, being an adult woman in these times is tough.

In previous centuries, women's clothing was altered to fit the person; now, we alter ourselves to fit clothing. While of course we do not want to return to the corsets and petticoats of previous eras, our only options now are to have ourselves snipped, tucked, rolled, dieted, and exercised into impossible shapes, just to suit the one-size-fits-all realities of mass-produced clothing.

Now, magazines, movies, social media, news, medical standards, fad diets, gurus, friends, relatives, and hordes of other sources try to tell us the "right" way to seek happiness, and for many of us, happiness is found in the ideal body size.

Of course, the "ideal" body size is right around size 0. Even our clothing sizes are skewed against us; it is literally impossible to look like a model without Photoshop. And yet, thousands of women every day do everything they can to be as thin, muscular, flawless, and made-over as the airbrushed images we see in magazines and online.

Education, media, politics, social media, and other societal factors continue to teach us who to be and how to be; by our 20s, we are often using diets, pills, exercise plans, nutrition gimmicks, expert advice, and any other system we can get our hands on in order to achieve our "ideal" self, which we have been downloading since birth.

Fashion models, by the way, are the highest-risk category for eating disorders for this exact reason: no one looks like the women in the pictures. Cindy Crawford, the model and actress, was asked how to "look like Cindy Crawford?" She responded, "I wish I looked like Cindy Crawford!" She meant that *no one* looked like Cindy Crawford, because the Cindy Crawford from pictures and movies simply does not exist. No one looks like that – it is all created by computer.

Not only do we see impossible celebrity examples of beauty, we see touched-up pictures of our friends and family on social media, where people only display themselves at their best. We judge others on their highlight reel and ourselves on the bloopers.

Hopelessness sets in as we strive for unrealistic expectations; society might as well tell us to chop off some toes for a smaller shoe size, for all the good it will do.

As we grow older, we are taught to look younger and younger (ironically). Men are often praised for aging – we call them "silver foxes" and other attractive nicknames. Women, by contrast, are sold products that promise to shed years from our lives, including Botox, creams, and other expensive, artificial interventions that can only prolong the inevitable.

In our 20s and 30s, we are sold all kinds of beauty products to make us the "ideal" body type; in our 40s and 50s, we are taught that we must look 20 or 30 again.

Asking a 40-year-old woman to look 20 is like asking a beautiful oak tree to force itself back into an acorn. It's ridiculous, cruel, and physically impossible. And yet, society asks us to change ourselves every single day, usually through buying a product or punishing ourselves through starvation and exercise.

Not only is this unrealistic, it is unfair. You are born with certain characteristics, such as your shoe size and eye color. Even those are criticized by society, who wants to sell you more ways to be thinner, look taller, have more energy. Aging is a beautiful, natural process, designed to move you through the various phases of life into your golden years.

During mid-life, women also experience hormonal changes that add further challenges. Fluctuating estrogen levels during perimenopause and menopause change our bodily rhythms that we have become accustomed to, altering our weight, our emotional state, adding extra stress, and generally wreaking havoc on our bodies.

So, while we are busy trying to wrangle ourselves into impossible shapes, we still have to maintain the other demands of life, including jobs, family responsibilities, and other stresses. You probably find yourself constantly taking care of others: your children, your children's children, your pets, your neighbors, your friends, your co-workers, your job, your house, your car, and then, of course, you have to carve out time for yourself in order to meet your health and fitness goals. There are only 24 hours in a day, after all, and sometimes those are just not enough.

In our culture, women are taught to sacrifice their own wellbeing for the wellbeing of others. Women over 40, in particular, often spend hours every day caring for others before they care for themselves.

Although your service is valuable and needed, how much do you do for others simply because that's the way it's always been? There is a big difference between "assisting" and "pleasing." Pleasing others is not truly helping them, it's just attempting to keep them from being mad at you. Trust me, it won't work.

If you've ever bent over backward to try and make someone's life better, only to have them criticize, belittle, and complain about the job you did, you know what I'm talking about.

Patterns of pleasing are passed down through generations, from times when it was considered inappropriate for women to work outside the home. In previous eras, one spouse in a household worked outside the home, and the other was left to take care of the cooking, cleaning, childcare, and other home-based chores.

In earlier times, communities of women tended to come together more often to share in household and outdoor chores, and women would spend time together watching each other's children and completing tasks together. By dividing up the work, there was less work to go around and more sharing in the benefits, even though their chores were harder, and they had more work to complete on a given day just to accomplish basic survival.

Times have changed, obviously. Now, women are able to have their own careers and goals and dreams, which is so necessary and important. Being able to do more is one of the greatest blessings of our era.

And yet, women are still largely expected to maintain the household chores. Some households are divided equitably, of course, but women are often asked to be the organizer of household chores even if they do not complete them on their own.

These days, we are left to accomplish everything ourselves, and our "labor saving" devices actually require more work from us, as they "free" us up to do more daily tasks. Instead of sharing the labor of childcare, cooking, cleaning, and other work, we are expected to handle them alone and considered weak if we ask for help.

Further, women are also asked to do a great deal of emotional labor to support and sustain their family and friend groups. Women, much more than men, are expected to listen and nurture in relationships and keep people feeling happy. This is a wonderful gift that many of us possess, but it can be a burden at times.

Still, we are certainly much better off than women of the past: women have claimed more opportunities than ever before. We do not have to put in long hours of physical labor to meet our fundamental necessities, and we have many conveniences that make our lives much simpler than in previous times. So why aren't we happy?

We claim more rights, equality, and abilities than in almost any other time.

We are granted access to our dreams, and many of us fulfill them each and every day.

However, not everyone stops to consider the costs of being able to do so many things. Being allowed to do so much sometimes mean you are required to do too much. We face a variety of social pressures that insist that because we can do *anything,* we have to do *everything.*

Doing everything is simply impossible. We often face pressure from others and from ourselves to be, do, have, and create everything we can, but there are only 24 hours in the day. It is simply impossible to maintain the modern lifestyle without sharing the work more evenly. Women are typically asked to do the work of many, alone.

Naturally, this is a problem.

Overtaxing yourself leads to burnout, stress, and chronic illness. If your only "me time" right now is the time you spend exercising to make yourself match impossible beauty standards, you actually don't have any "me time" at all – you are spending that time trying to please others.

Of course, we can and should leave our mark on Earth; each of us has a purpose and we must do our best to fulfill it. In fact, we are all here on this planet to help others, but there comes a point when helping is actually just enabling. You can't make everyone happy, so quit trying.

In fact, if you are sacrificing your own health and wellbeing in an attempt to be acceptable to others, you are likely doing them a disservice. Although it might make their life easier right now, it ultimately harms them in the long run because they have not learned to care for themselves.

People-pleasing is actually a form of manipulation. If you have to fawn all over other people to keep them from whining, throwing tantrums, or acting out, you are actually allowing their own immature behavior to continue by feeding it. Your own behavior is also immature, because mature behavior means allowing others to own their choices. Resorting to manipulation is not a true form of power: it is weakness. In the meantime, no one is happy.

Not only is people pleasing weak and manipulative, overtaxing yourself to please others is dangerous to your health *and* the health of those you are trying to please. It's much harder to help people from a hospital bed, which is where you will be sooner or later if you do not take control of your own health. In fact, the people you are trying to help now will then be required to take care of you, which might feel like sweet revenge in the moment, but ultimately only hurts you.

Regaining your vitality will allow you to help those around you even more by finding your best self. When you are stronger, happier, and healthier, you will be able to do so much more for yourself and the others around you.

You will be better able to lend support when you yourself have the resources you need to thrive; on airplanes, we are told to put the oxygen mask on ourselves before assisting others. No one can save anyone's life if they are themselves gasping for air. It's time for a metaphorical oxygen mask.

You're not "over the hill," you are entering the prime of life – your best years are ahead of you.

If you believe that your life is all downhill from here, you have been lied to. Limiting beliefs like these serve no one, especially because they are blatant falsehoods.

For an example of someone who refused to let aging get the better of her, just look at Ernestine Shepherd, who began training as a bodybuilder at age 71. If it were impossible, she wouldn't have done it!

Everyone can be like Ernestine, if they choose to be – even you.

Although you cannot stop yourself from growing older, you can stop yourself from growing old. Aging is a natural process of life; being elderly is optional.

If weight and other health issues are getting in your way, it's time to take a closer look at your life and let go of what no longer serves you. If you have spent decades in soul-crushing jobs, abusive relationships, numbing your feelings, addictions, drama, or other issues that you just can't seem to shake, your weight is simply there to protect you from feeling the deeper feelings. It's time to look your problems in the face, give them a big "thank you!" and send them on their way.

This book will teach you strategies to gain back some control over your life by focusing on all four dimensions of wellbeing: mental, emotional, spiritual, and physical. By tapping into all four, you can learn to be fit, fun, and fierce again at *any* age, despite what you might have been taught about what it means to be a woman over 40.

To become the fit and fabulous you that you deserve to be, you can work on your mental and emotional patterns, which are the foundation for all your physical realities.

As the saying goes, we are not physical beings having a spiritual experience, but spiritual beings having a physical experience. All physical issues have an underlying cause rooted in mental, emotional, or spiritual needs.

Think about the last time you binged on something that wasn't good for you – was it a physical need? Or an emotional one? Chances are good that you filled a physical hole in an attempt to fill a deeper hole in your soul; fill the hole, and the craving goes away.

Our mental, emotional, spiritual, and physical states are so entwined that we cannot always tell the difference. We resort to physical-world changes because it's the part of our reality that we can see, hear, smell, taste, and touch.

Remember the last time you cried? You experienced physical sensations, such as tears and breath-pattern changes, but you also experienced emotional, mental, and spiritual sensations that might be harder to put into words. Still, they were there. Crying is a good example of the ways our physical body is synonymous with our mental, emotional, and spiritual selves, but it's not the only example. Laughing, dancing, and other autonomous behaviors also operate on all four levels, and each level affects the other. It's a reciprocal relationship.

In the same way, health is not just physical: it is also mental, emotional, and spiritual. If you have imbalances in other areas of your life, your physical self will cry out for help. These cries come in the form of weight issues, illness, fatigue, and other common aging symptoms.

If you are reading this, chances are you have tried countless health and nutrition programs trying to lose weight. These kinds of solutions might work temporarily, of course, if you have enough discipline, but sooner or later, the weight returns. The underlying unease and vague dissatisfaction probably never left. It was there all along, just below the surface, waiting to come crashing back the moment you re-gained even a pound.

That is partly why the weight always comes back – you never changed the patterns that kept you from losing the weight and keeping it off.

You are not alone. The health and fitness industry is a multi-billion dollar business for a reason – everyone is eager to try the latest fad, the newest plan to achieve the fleeting happiness of the next big diet or workout.

Physical approaches ultimately fail because they only focus on one dimension of health. If you find yourself trying solution after solution only to end up dissatisfied, try starting with the other three dimensions first. Physical changes will quickly follow, and they will be natural, gentle, and safe. Your body knows what it needs. It knows better than you do, in fact, and it knows infinitely more than a diet pill, slim-down-fast scheme, or shiny workout package.

Using this book's integrated approach, you can change those underlying patterns and allow your body to naturally regain its vitality for a fitter, more fun, fiercer you.

So far, I have discussed societal factors leading to body dissatisfaction, which, ironically, also leads us to gain and keep weight (which is convenient for diet pill companies, isn't it?). Society's pressures to lose weight actually keep us heavier due to the emotional toll they take on us, so those pressures are the first things to go when you begin any serious attempt to change your life. Still, I need to dedicate the rest of this chapter to something you might not always connect with weight: trauma.

If you are like every member of the human family, you experienced trauma in childhood. That trauma is likely still with you, holding you back from reaching your highest potential. Now, some of us experience serious trauma through abuse, neglect, serious injury or accident, or other deeply scarring incidents in our childhoods and adulthoods. Those are significant, powerful events that must be dealt with before any true healing can begin.

However, all of us experience at least some level of trauma, whether we realize it or not. Infancy, childhood, and teen years are filled with conflict, illness, injury, and other stressors that stay with us much longer than we realize. Your body remembers everything that has ever happened to you, whether or not you can recall it in your mind's eye.

In your earliest days, you were learning what it meant to be a human being and how to get along as a member of your family and friend groups. As a young person, you had very little control, so you learned to cope by avoiding triggers or lashing out. When anything unpleasant happened, your body filed that way as a silent reminder of how not to get hurt again, and you either withdrew or fought back. Bullies, shouting relatives, loud teachers, global conflicts, and other uncontrollable situations left their mark on you, and you did whatever felt right to keep yourself safe.

Trauma-learned patterns are still with you, and manifest themselves in your relationships, your work, your habits, your beliefs, and indeed, your whole life. As just one example, if you are afraid of dogs and believe men are manipulative, you learned that through experience, before you can even remember. In your experience, dogs are aggressive, men are manipulative. This pattern has proven itself true over and over with every new dog and man you meet. Even if you have a twin sister who loves dogs and adores men, you cannot – you have learned that it's impossible.

If you take an inventory of your most firmly held beliefs, you probably can trace them back to something you learned from a childhood trauma. The example of dogs and men is just one way that the world might be tinted through the lens of trauma: maybe you believe that nothing ever works out for you or that you never make any money, no matter how hard you try.

Or, more pertinently, maybe you believe that no matter how much you diet, you can never lose weight. Perhaps as a baby, toddler, or small child you were told that you were "chunky," or had "adorable fat cheeks," so you keep those patterns to live up to your family's expectations. Maybe you were pinched and prodded and grabbed whenever you were thin, so putting on some weight kept you from being taken advantage of by others. You likely don't remember this, but your body does.

Of course, some of these patterns were learned in other ways. Your own mother (or maternal caregiver) left her mark on you, biologically and socially. In your earliest days, you perceived yourself as essentially the same person as your mother as a residual connection from the umbilical cord, and later on, her mood directly affected your ability to get the food, sleep, and care you needed because she was the one who provided it. Any anger, stress, grief, or other troubles she experienced became yours.

To a certain extent, that bond is likely still with you, even if you haven't spoken to your mother in years or even if she is no longer living. Any beliefs that your family members held about weight or body image or beauty are firmly rooted in your psyche. You will need to root them out.

The lessons you learned between birth and the age of three were the foundational beliefs of your life. Your family taught you a number of underlying beliefs without even realizing it, and they did this to keep you safe. However, those beliefs might no longer be necessary. In fact, they might actually be holding you back.

Your mother's and other family member's experiences are your experiences, whether you like it or not. To some extent, this is part of life, but acknowledging this is the first step to becoming your own person.

Of course, your mother (and other people) had no idea how their experiences affected you. Parents and teachers are just trying their best and were in turn traumatized by their own parents and teachers; the vicious cycle extends through the generations.

In an ideal world, parents and caregivers would be physically, emotionally, mentally, and spiritually healthy, fully capable of providing themselves and others with unconditional love and care. Teachers and playmates would be joyful and loving, and we would all support each other in becoming our highest and best selves.

Unfortunately, ours is not an ideal world. Parents are people, too, and by the time we get out of school, most (if not all) of us have experienced trauma to one degree or another. These traumas might be big or small, but we all experienced sadness, fear, worry, loss, and other traumatizing events as young children. Women, in particular, face physical forms of trauma throughout their lives and carry it as extra weight, and many of us have experienced serious traumas that can be debilitating.

For many of us, dealing with trauma means turning to unhealthy coping mechanisms: bingeing, over-exercise, under-exercise, crash diets, addictions, and other attempts to take control of the terrible things that have happened to us. As we age, these troubles tend to worsen. The drinks and foods we can easily handle in our 20s quickly become obsessive nightmares as we crave, cave, and then hate ourselves; the cycle then repeats to infinity. Other solutions are necessary in order to deal with whatever traumas you still carry.

One solution to healing trauma is forgiveness, but you are not required to forgive anyone else's behavior unless you are fully ready to do so – they made choices that now affect you, and you have every right to be angry.

Still, spending precious time and energy blaming perpetrators only hurts you more. Perpetrators, too, were carrying trauma and unleashed it on others because they knew no other way to live. The perpetrators of trauma also carry trauma, which they received from perpetrators who were also carrying trauma, and so the vicious cycle continues.

It is up to us to break the chain by letting go of our own stake in that trauma. Breaking the chain does not necessarily mean forgiving the perpetrator, though. For now, a simple acceptance that your trauma is not your fault might be enough.

If you are unsure if trauma is a factor in your life, open yourself to the possibility that your health and fitness might be caused by something that is not your fault. It's easy to place the blame elsewhere: on genetics, on carbs, on medications, or any other number of factors. And while those physical elements certainly play a significant role, look at all the people who live the same kind of lifestyle with no adverse effects. Those people have either dealt with their trauma, were lucky enough to experience less trauma than you, or carry their trauma in different ways – sooner or later, everyone's trauma catches up to them.

If you were led to this book, it's because you are ready to begin laying that trauma down and healing, once and for all.

Have you ever felt like crying after a deep tissue massage or intense yoga class? That is because trauma is stored in your physical cells and can be released in deep relaxation. Once you have allowed your trauma to heal, you can easily shed any excess pounds; more importantly, you will feel happier, freer, and more able to live your truest and best self.

As I mentioned previously, I experienced several traumatizing challenges that impacted me deeply. Particularly, a few years ago I was homeless, pregnant, and going through a divorce due to domestic violence. My young son and I lived in a homeless shelter for almost two years. The challenges we face may be different, but the wherewithal needed to get through them is the same.

Everyone experiences trials, tribulations, challenges, or whatever you prefer to call it. It's what we do in those times that affect who we become. I remember a time of desperation and wanting change. I saw a fork in my road: either do what's best for my wellbeing, or not. For me, the choice was between dealing with the occasional drunk, angry husband just for the sake of having a marriage and a two-parent household, even when he's in denial and won't get help, or leaving and finding my own path. I asked myself, *do I continue to deal with the tension, anxiety, and stress affecting my wellbeing and the wellbeing of my child? Or do I make the changes necessary to move my life forward?*

So, I'm asking you: are you going to continue to make excuses and deal with something you don't want? I had to take a deep dive into myself to stay focused on accomplishing my goals.

I had to apply the same determination and drive to get out of that situation that you will need to change your situation. I know you have it within you, or you would not be reading this book right now. If you combine the three major elements that control your wellbeing, you will feel amazing and soon will see physical improvements. Not only will you look and feel younger, but your biological age will also reverse on the cellular level. You will enjoy new vitality, a newly found empowerment, and a greater sense of freedom. You will feel well about yourself. Every single day you will be getting closer to the dynamic state of wholeness.

Many people have thanked me for how my work has changed their life, allowing them to feel satisfaction, happiness, and vibrancy for the first time after years of suffering. You can experience the same success and feel better by applying the knowledge contained in this book.

Ultimately, the only person who can choose to change your life is you. You can work with other people, get the help you need, incorporate a variety of techniques, but the only person who can actually take the first step is you. After the first step, don't stop until you have reached your full potential.

No matter who you are, where you are, or what your history is, you can use this same process to achieve a healthier, happier you. There is no better time than right now.

This book will teach you crucial steps you can take on the path to improving your health and wellness. I'm glad you have decided to join me on the journey.

This book takes you through the mind, body, and spirit dimensions of wellness to help you become fit and fabulous at any age. You can regain your vitality and make your later years your best years.

This book first shows you...

1. How to harness your mind for greater willpower and strength in your fitness goals.
2. How to recalibrate your body for optimum health and wellness.
3. How your spirit (your beliefs, values, dreams, and emotions) can be harnessed to launch you to reach your highest potential.

Chapter 1

Wholeness & Wellness

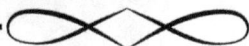

$\sim\!\!\diamond\!\!\sim$

I f you look around the world today, you will see a vast majority of people who are *re*active, rather than *pro*active. Living a joyful life means taking responsibility for what happens; although you might not have been the cause of your circumstances, you are the one who is ultimately responsible for your choices. Taking ownership of your life is the most powerful step you can take.

None of us can control our circumstances. What you can control, however, is what you make of the circumstances you are given. You can complain until you are blue in the face, but not one ounce of change will occur until you get up and *do* something about it.

Please remember that you are not responsible for any abuse, neglect, ill treatment, diseases, inherited traits, or anything else that might be a challenge for you. Each of us is given a particular set of challenges to overcome, and most (if not all) of the time we do not have direct control over what happens to us. However, there is one person who can take those challenges and turn them into successes: you.

The best we can do is to take the cards we were handed by Fate, God, the Universe, whatever you want to call it, and make the best of them. I trust that you will choose the road to empowerment. Empowered people might not like the cards they have been dealt, but they choose to take those cards and play them as best they can. They don't blame their parents, their family, the schools, capitalism, the government, or the heavens for their misfortune and for what they are experiencing in that moment. They assume full responsibility for themselves and their life.

To make a personalized plan to tackle your specific situation and take informed, conscious action, you need to first observe yourself and your life carefully. The following self-assessment will ask you some tough questions about your current outlook. Fair warning: self-assessment can get uncomfortable, but it is necessary. Life is already uncomfortable, and the quickest way out is through. You are taking a brave step, but the results are worth it.

SELF-ASSESSMENT EXERCISE

Find a silent spot where you can spend some time pondering your answers.

YOUR BODY

What is your ideal weight?_____

What is your current weight? _____

How much would you like to lose? _____

Jot down your relationship with weight. Use the following questions to guide you:

What is your relationship with weight?:

Have you always had weight problems? If your weight has been fluctuating, what did you do to lose weight and what happened when you regained the lost weight?

Do you eat more than you ate when you were at your ideal weight? Have you changed your eating habits in any way? Frequency of eating, cooking less, more prepared food, or eating junk food, or drinking sugary drinks, etc.? Do you have any food addictions? Do you have any food cravings?

_____

_____

_____

_____

_____

_____

_____

_____

_____

_____

It is 3:00 in the morning. You just got out of bed and walked into the kitchen. You open your fridge and take out something to eat. What is it?

_____

_____

Things are not going well. You feel sad, worried, and depressed. What do you want to eat? _____

_____

If you work out, how often? _____

How long?_____

How many times per week? _____

On a scale from 1 to 10, how fit are you? _____

Have you changed your workout habits since you started to gain weight?

_____

YOUR EMOTIONS

On a scale from 1 to 10, how stressed out are you on a typical day?

_____

What people, events, things, and situations cause you stress? How do you react to and deal with them?

_____

_____

_____

_____

What is your habitual emotional state? _____

_____

You wake up in the morning. Your eyes open. What is your first thought and your first feeling?

_____

_____

_____

_____

_____

Walk up to a mirror and with as neutral a face as possible take a good look at your face. Look at all the features separately. Does your "neutral" face reflect any suppressed emotions? Do you look sad, angry, tired, doubtful, disgusted, worried, etc.?

_____

_____

_____

_____

_____

Do you hold grudges? If yes, what are the triggers?

_____

_____

_____

_____

Do you live in fear? Do you do or not do things because you are afraid something bad will happen if you do or if you don't?

_____

_____

_____

_____

_____

Do you communicate your feelings and emotions clearly to others or do you hold them back?

_____

_____

_____

_____

_____

What is your emotional state when you habitually choose to eat comfort food? _____

_____

_____

_____

_____

Look back to your past and list the most typical feelings and emotions you have experienced, especially since and right before you started to gain weight. Now write down how you really feel about yourself, your body, your emotional and mental state, your success, your relationships, your career, your love life, your aspirations, your creativity, your purpose and mission in life. Don't hold back! Write until you have nothing more left to write.

_____

_____

_____

_____

_____

_____

_____

_____

_____

_____

_____

_____

_____

_____

_____

_____

_____

_____

_____

_____

_____

_____

YOUR MENTAL STATE

In life we go through phases where the majority of our thoughts, feelings and emotions lean more on either the positive side or the negative side. Our negative side contributes to the decline in health and wellness.

We must recognize it and become aware of it so we can stop it and put forth the effort to change it. (If a question goes not apply to you, simply writ in N/A)

Finish the following sentences according to what you believe. Don't overthink it. Don't try to override your unconscious beliefs by saying something that you know you should think of yourself but you actually think something else. Doing so would defeat the purpose of this discovery exercise. You are searching for the hidden, unconscious programs and beliefs, so whatever comes to your mind first, jot it down immediately. Do not filter anything. Use the space below to fill in each sentence as it relates to your wellbeing:

Life is _____

_____

_____

I am _____

_____

_____

I am unlovable because _____

_____

I am ugly and _____

because _____

I am fat and _____

_____

I deserve to be punished because _____

_____

I deserve to be fat and unhealthy because _____

_____

I am powerless and _____

_____

I am too _____

to create the life I want. _____

I am too _____

to lose weight. _____

I deserve a _____

life because _____

Beautiful women are _____

_____

Women who have a strong, healthy body are _____

_____

Fat women are _____

_____

Middle aged women are _____

_____

Men are _____

_____

I cannot trust _____

because _____

I cannot be trusted because _____

_____

I am too tired to _____

_____

I don't deserve _____

because _____

If I will lose weight and be slim, men will _____

_____

If I will lose weight and be slim, women will _____

_____

If I will lose weight and be slim, my mother will _____

_____

If I will lose weight and be slim, my father will _____

_____

If I will be strong and fit, people will _____

_____

It pays to be overweight and unattractive because _____

_____

If I will be strong and fit, my life will _____

and I can't let that happen. _____

I'm afraid that if I lose weight and be fit and strong _____

_____

On a scale of 1-10, how willing are you to take the reins of your life and get fit and fabulous? _____

_____

On a scale of 1-10, how scared are you to take the reins of your life and get fit and fabulous? _____

_____

Now that you have finished the assessment, take a minute to check in with yourself. How do you feel?

If you're feeling uncomfortable, don't worry. Self-assessment can be difficult, as we often have to face up to harsh truths. However, that's the beauty of it – understanding ourselves is the first and most necessary step.

This kind of work takes effort. We feel uncomfortable with this kind of inner work because our ego tells us not to rock the boat. We have clichés that teach us things like, "you can't teach an old dog new tricks," meaning that once a person is set in their ways, they can never change.

Research on personality used to argue that a person was set in their ways by age 30, but recent research has proven that that is false. We can change our personality at any age, and we can also change our habits.

Not only can we change our habits, we can literally change our mental patterns, which in turn changes the literal makeup of our brains. Research into neuroplasticity is proving that humans can think new thoughts and build new neural pathways. Our brains build "ruts" as we think similar thoughts over time, building up a "path of least resistance." Although it can be hard to move our brains out of the rut (just like a wheelbarrow taken over the same track over and over again), once we build a newer, better rut, the brain takes to it very well.

If you start to change your mental patterns, your brain will start to dig new "ruts" in your newer, better way of thinking. It will take time, but it will happen.

At first, it will feel uncomfortable. Lean into this discomfort. Everything is hard at first, as I'm sure you remember from childhood when you started school or learned to ride a bike. It got easier, but it took time. Building your new life will require similar dedication and patience, but it will be worth it.

First, though, what does your ideal life look like? The pursuit of happiness, after all, is based in arbitrary standards about what your life is supposed to look like compared to everyone else around you. Now, it's time to discover what your own life *could* look like by tapping into your inner self.

Your heart holds your deepest desires. However, our heart's true desires rarely match what you have been taught you *should* want. We are taught to want a big house, 2.5 kids, a husband, an SUV, a six-figure job, exotic vacations, and all kinds of tangible markers of success. These things are fine to have, if they are truly making you happy. So many of us have these things but fail to actually enjoy them, because there is something else missing: true love for ourselves and our life.

Although material success is wonderful, exciting, and even attainable, if you listen to your heart carefully, it might whisper that there are other things you want more than physical abundance.

Your heart is probably craving abundance on the mental, emotional, and spiritual levels of your being. Perhaps you want true connection with a partner or the ability to truly perfect your skills and talents. Maybe you have been craving adventure or education or something that seems impossible in your current financial or physical situation. You might have always wanted to start your own business or write a book or change the world in some way. Until you achieve (or at least pursue) your innermost desires, no house or car or family or vacation will ever fill that hole.

Once you shut off the relentless chatter about how you and your life *should* be, you will be free to follow your true desires and find real joy, contentment, and happiness.

After you focus on your heart's desires, you can still seek the big house and fancy clothes and dream vacation if you want them. In fact, you might have the chance for *more* of those things, if your dreams include them.

More importantly, though, you will be more satisfied with them. Your daily life will excite you, and you will gain enjoyment in the everyday. You will feel like you are "enough," and the comments, attitudes, and possessions of other people will not feel personal anymore. You will be a self-contained vessel, impervious to the actions of others.

So, it's time to contact the real you, the one who is beyond the external expectations and hidden deep inside. She has been waiting for you. She might even surprise you with her abilities, talents, skills, desires, dreams, and goals.

Do this exercise when you can set aside at least an hour to focus without interruptions. If you can be completely alone and in nature, even better. If that's not possible, find a nature sound recording and play it during the exercise. Nature sounds will help you put your brain into an alpha state where your conscious mind steps back and you can more easily get in touch with your unconscious mind.

We often suppress our true desires because our cultural beliefs and programs tell us that it is not right to go after them. Not following your heart causes pain and suffering, so we unconsciously "forget" what we would really like to do, have, or be. We gradually bury our true desires so that we do not have to feel again the pain of not seeing them come true.

EXERCISE: IMAGINING YOUR PERFECT LIFE

It is time to get back into contact with your heart (your true self) and find out what it is that you may have forgotten. Grab a pen (do not use digital devices for this exercise) and spend a few minutes just breathing and listening to yourself. Remember how you felt when you were a child and used to daydream? Without trying to filter things out for being "ridiculous," "unattainable," "illogical," or just "not for you. If after an hour you feel stuck, move on and come back to these pages whenever new ideas pop up.

How do I really want my life to be like 1 year from now?

Date: _____

Health & Fitness:

_____

_____

_____

_____

_____

_____

Work:

_____

_____

_____

_____

_____

_____

Relationship:

_____

_____

_____

_____

_____

_____

Life's Mission:

_____

_____

_____

_____

_____

_____

_____

Personal Growth Goals:

_____

_____

_____

_____

_____

_____

Wanted Experiences:

_____

_____

_____

_____

_____

_____

How do I really want my life to be like in 3 years from now?

Date: _____

Health & Fitness:

_____

_____

_____

_____

_____

_____

Work:

_____

_____

_____

_____

_____

Relationship:

_____

_____

_____

_____

_____

Life's Mission:

_____

_____

_____

_____

_____

_____

_____

Personal Growth Goals:

_____

_____

_____

_____

_____

_____

Wanted Experiences:

_____

_____

_____

_____

_____

_____

Imagine all the beliefs that no longer serve you written on pieces of paper. Mentally take these imaginary pieces of paper and imagine yourself putting them in a suitcase and snapping it shut. See yourself handing that suitcase back to the people or places that gave you those negative beliefs while mentally saying to those people and places, "these belong to you, so I am returning them to you now." Then, never take those beliefs back. Repeat this exercise as often as necessary.

In this book we will concentrate on transforming you into your fit and fabulous self, but it is important that you have a full picture of what you truly want because our body image, and eating issues, which most of the time are strongly tied in to us not living the life we would really like to live.

In the rest of the book we will tackle fitness and health, but if you start with your inner needs first, the outer needs will follow more easily. In fact, you will find yourself eager, able, and ready to attend to physical needs because the inner needs have already been met. The results might astound you.

Now that you completed your self-discovery it time to apply it to action. To change your mind, body, and spirit...

1. For any negative thoughts or beliefs you still carry about yourself and your weight, change them to a positive affirmation of your fitness goals.
2. Believe that it's possible. See it as already done.
3. Feel the emotions you have as a new person – the person you are already becoming.

CHAPTER 2

THE ART OF VITALITY

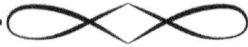

Our bodies are magnificent, complex systems. They breathe, pump blood, avoid danger, manage stress, grow, heal, and thousands of other functions without our conscious knowledge. Our instinctive knowledge, partly gained from experience and learning and partly innately born within us, keeps us functioning, sometimes even in spite of ourselves.

However, we are also capable of conscious engagement with these automated behaviors. Just as we can decide how deep or shallow a breath to take, we can take control of our subconscious patterns and habits. In time, they become our new unconscious.

Having this capability means that we are responsible for the kind of life we live. We have a choice, every single minute of every single day, how we want to live.

When I refer to *vitality*, I mean more than just being alive. Vitality comes from the Latin root *vita*, which means "life." Truly *living* means to both consciously and unconsciously choose life over death.

To be living, instead of merely existing, requires a conscious exercise of will. Similar to the difference between automatic breathing and conscious breathing, there is also a difference between the unconscious sustenance of the physical body and the (conscious or unconscious) mental choice to choose life over death. Let me explain.

Vitality has a nutritional element, which means that if you feed your body with the optimal whole foods and exercise it regularly according to its capabilities and needs (by training, walking and moving around in your day-to-day), your body will remain in an optimal shape and state of fitness.

Animals in the wild do not need self-help books to maintain vitality. They maintain a species-specific diet simply by following their instincts and foraging for whatever food is available. An animal never weighs the nutritional value of two plants in order to choose which one to eat – it will decide instinctively, without even thinking about it. And animals do not binge (although some domesticated animals will, if given free reign of processed, manufactured feed).

Humans, of course, are different. We exist in complex, multi-layered systems of information, access, and beliefs about food, and we must navigate them every minute of every day. In previous eras, circumstances were different, by and large, and access to food was often a serious problem.

Now, certain areas of the planet struggle to access food, but the other areas suffer the opposite problem – too many choices.

Because humans no longer live in our natural rural habitats, our eating habits are completely removed from our evolved nutritional needs. This gap is growing more evident every year, made more obvious by the thousands of books written on nutrition and the fact that scientists don't seem to agree about what constitutes a natural human diet. Isn't it ironic that we consider ourselves the most intelligent species on Earth, and yet, we seem to be unable to agree on what we should eat?

The shifting diets of the human species means that we learned to love food that tastes good, rather than what is healthy for us. Over time, we have forgotten what species-specific eating means for the human body. Our bodies have gotten so used to unnatural, highly processed foods and strange food combinations that we have lost our intuitive abilities to sense the foods we need.

The more humans eat foods that are not naturally meant for humans to eat (e.g., artificial sweeteners, processed sugar, processed grains, etc.), the more the body gets overloaded by toxins and other substances that add stressors on our body systems. As we age, we become more and more susceptible to imbalances in the gut, causing further complications.

Recent research has taught us that your cravings are actually not feeding you – they're feeding your microbiome. The microbiome is the complex environment of beneficial and harmful bacteria that lives in and on every human, animal, plant, surface, and the whole planet. Humans have a specific microbiome that must be in balance for optimum health. Increasingly, processed foods, chemicals, stress, poor health, and other factors throw off this balance. In fact, your cravings are largely driven by the bacteria in your gut, rather than your own needs.

In particular, the human biome needs a healthy balance between good bacteria and bad bacteria to function properly. "Good" and "bad" refers to the extent to which each bacterial strain is beneficial or harmful; for instance, *candida albicans* is one strain of bacteria that is labeled "bad," but each of us have and need this strain, to some extent.

The trouble comes when it gets out of whack, which we call candida overgrowth. Candida, by the way, loves to eat carbs. Ring any bells?

So, your cravings for carbs, sugar, junk food, processed snacks, and other goodies might not even be coming from you. You can blame the bacteria. However, that doesn't mean you are off the hook: bacterial overgrowth can cause all kinds of issues, as the waste products of harmful bacteria can lead to toxicity, inflammation, and other serious problems if allowed to run rampant.

Some people believe *all* bacteria is bad, but this could not be further from the truth. Bacteria is inevitable, and we need good bacteria to thrive. In fact, a healthy microbiome includes trillions of beneficial bacteria, which are responsible for our overall wellbeing. The byproducts of "good" bacteria assist with the creation of hormones (such as serotonin, the "feel-good molecule").

When beneficial bacteria succumb to harmful bacteria and the balance is thrown off, our gut health suffers. Our gut health is integral to our overall wellbeing; in fact, scientists are beginning to refer to the gut as the "second brain." When parasites overcome the good bugs in our systems, they secrete chemicals that send cravings to our brains. We then eat more bread, pasta, and corn flakes, feeding the bacteria, who grow and send out more cravings. Then, the vicious cycle continues.

Beneficial bacteria thrive on whole, natural foods. Prebiotic foods feed beneficia bacteria and probiotic foods contain beneficial bacteria, so you need those in abundance.

You must also do your best, however, to limit foods that harm beneficial bacteria. Antibiotics, too, are highly dangerous to beneficial bacteria, as antibiotics are generic and do not discriminate between the good and the bad.

If you have taken antibiotics often in your life, eaten the Standard American Diet (SAD), or have frequent digestive issues, your gut biome probably needs a little tender, loving care. For full health and vitality, we must feed our tiny, invisible friends the microbes. Trust me, they will thank you for it.

In previous eras, people ate fermented (probiotic) foods regularly. It was the most common way to preserve food before widespread refrigeration. Their bread, too, was prepared using the fermentation process (what we now call sourdough bread) instead of using the instant yeast packets and sugar of today.

All so-called "primitive" cultures now have maintained their traditional methods for preparing food, and these cultures are actually much healthier than eaters of the Standard American Diet (SAD). Ancient diets were more efficient, less wasteful, and made better use of the nutrients found in food.

For instance, another difference between recent and ancient humans was their tendency to use the entire animal when eating animal products. Instead of using just the choicest meats and throwing the rest away, as we do now, they used the entire animal, including the bones. The recent bone broth craze is based in this idea of waste and rooted in research that demonstrates that your gut needs a variety of vitamins and minerals to thrive, including the minerals found in the wasted parts of animals. Our soil and water is depleted of essential minerals today, so bone broth is one way that we can replenish some of those missing nutrients and revitalize your gut, which needs adequate minerals to work properly.

Probiotics, in fact, make vitamins and minerals more bioavailable because they assist the body in breaking down the particles of food as you digest. The widespread increase in lactose intolerance today has much to do with the way that pasteurized, homogenized milk has lost the beneficial bacteria found in raw milk, which assists the stomach in breaking it down. Many people who get sick from store-bought milk do fine on raw milk straight from the cow because the bacteria in raw milk assists their bodies in breaking it down. Of course, some people have serious lactose intolerance and you should always consult with a doctor about your individual needs.

We also have a tendency to hyper-sanitize our food, our homes, and our bodies. Although cleanliness is important, stripping our environments of crucial bacteria actually throws our biomes out of balance. Babies have a tendency to eat dirt because their instincts let them know that bacteria is good for their immune system. Since modern humans live, work, and play in hyper-sanitized environments, we are lacking in thousands of tiny helpers that assist us in breaking down foods.

In former times, humans preserved food by pickling and fermenting and they had a tendency to use fermented foods as condiments with every meal. That way, whatever they ate, they digested it well and received as much benefit from it as possible, because their invisible bacterial friends were there to break down their food. The mild alcoholic drinks that humans used to consume regularly were actually fermented products that assisted with this process.

Alcohol, in fact, used to be made through a natural fermentation process that provided beneficial bacteria to the gut, but no longer. Modern processed alcohol does nothing for the gut but stress it out; eliminating alcohol from your diet as much as possible is an important step you can take to avoid filling yourself with extra calories and stress.

If you have indigestion, acid reflux, IBS, GERD, food allergies, intolerances, frequent bowel illnesses, or almost any other kind of digestive upset, it is likely that your gut biome needs assistance. Most modern Western people have these issues, and they contribute to a variety of other functional problems in the entire body.

To regain your vitality, it is imperative to eliminate addictive foods, detox, and nurture your gut biome. Believe it or not, it's not *how much* you are eating, it's *what* you are eating. You can eat plentiful amounts of nurturing foods and feel full and satisfied, if the foods you eat are actually contributing to vitality. The bacteria in your body are the ones who want to overeat, not you.

In particular, grains, carbohydrates, sugars, processed sugars, artificial sweeteners, and other treats are candida's favorite snacks. If you are now lamenting the loss of your entire diet, do not despair. Your cravings for these things are artificial, which means they are temporary. As you discipline yourself to avoid those foods and fill your diet with nutritious, supportive foods, those cravings will eventually leave on their own.

Supportive foods for your gut include probiotic, fermented foods, preferably made at home or bought directly from the person who fermented it; time spent on store shelves or in probiotic capsules is death to the tiny microbes. Still, if store-bought is all you can get, something is better than nothing. Fermented foods are actually simple to make and you can make them right on your kitchen counter with a few simple ingredients and a little time.

Some other powerful foods for your gut include anything that forms a "gel" – mucosal foods. These foods include aloe, flaxseeds, chia seeds, hemp seeds, bone broth, gelatin, and anything else that naturally gels up. The gel of these foods coats the lining of your intestines and helps to seal any permeability in your gut (also known as "leaky gut"), a common problem in modern humans.

Of course, you will want to find organic, non-GMO sources of these foods whenever possible and eat them in forms low in sugar. One way to eat seeds such as chia, flax, and hemp is to let them sit overnight in plenty your favorite dairy or non-dairy milk with some fruit. They will swell up into a gel-like "pudding" and fill up the container, so be sure to leave them extra room to grow. The "pudding" is full of healthy fats, minerals, vitamins, and is excellent for your gut.

As you can see, your efforts at changing your diet and your life will require consistent effort and significant adjustments to the way you live and work. Be patient with yourself, as these changes will take time. Changing your microbiome will change your body's ability to handle almost any food you can throw at it, giving you greater resilience, strength, and vitality.

Indeed, simply changing your diet alone will be a significant step on the path to vitality, before you even add exercise. You will want to get comfortable with a healthier diet as the foundation of your overall transformation.

The first change you need to make is with food, especially the kinds of food you are eating and when you are eating them. Food comes first; exercise is later. The *amount* of food is much less important than the *kind* of food you are eating. I cover exercise in another chapter, but food is much more important than you might think.

In the meantime, however, you must learn to develop willpower and change your diet to a healthier, more intuitive one. Change is difficult, and humans are creatures of comfort. We get used to certain foods because we have had them our whole lives and they make us feel good. Our taste buds struggle to like new things (although trying things over and over has been shown to acclimate us to them).

If you have tried dozens (or maybe even hundreds) of times to give up carbs or other foods and failed every time, know that this time is different. Before, you were trying to use sheer force of will, rather than knowledge.

Now, you can re-frame your perspective toward food and health and use your new outlook to develop willpower to make the changes you need to.

In fact, willpower is actually a replenishable resource. Previous research on willpower suggested that when you used it up, it was gone; newer research, however, is showing that willpower, like a muscle, can be exercised and grow with time. So, you can learn to replace your addictive usage of carbs with deliberate, meaningful usage of whole, wholesome foods by learning to develop willpower, which can grow in the same way your muscles develop when you go to the gym.

A major step in this process will be re-balancing your microbiome, which more than likely unbalanced. As you do, those candida-caused cravings will fade on their own.

To do this, you will need to feed your beneficial gut bacteria while eliminating everything that feeds harmful bacteria. There are a few ways you can do this, and you will need to use the one (or a combination of several) that works best for you.

Pick solutions that you can handle and commit to them.

The best solution is the one you will actually stick to; you can always add more solutions once you've mastered the first one, but now is the time to exercise your willpower muscles by choosing solutions that you are willing to see through to the end, and then sticking to it faithfully. It might be hard at first, as you pull yourself out of the mental "rut" you are in, but your new "ruts" will be absolutely worth it.

Our ancestors did not have the constant access to food that we do today. When the pre-modern person woke up in the morning, they had no certainty that there would be food, unless they went out to look for it in the wild. They had to constantly hunt and gather plants and animals to eat, and they often had to do it on an empty stomach.

Today, sugar has become our basic fuel, and we eat it on an almost-constant basis. The nice thing about sugar is that the energy is available almost immediately; however, it quickly depletes. When we eat carbohydrates (or even vegetables and meats, to a certain extent), the blood sugar spikes, giving us strength and vitality. The high quickly wears off, though, and we start to feel lightheaded, stressed, and hungry. We eat again, and the cycle continues.

Thankfully, our body contains a ketogenic system that provide an alternative fuel source for our body: ketones. When we have not eaten in a while, our liver starts to create ketones, which keep us going for a long time.

Intermittent fasting is one method that can be beneficial to starving out harmful bacteria. By eating as much as you want during certain hours of the day and then going without food for 13-15 hours per day, your body's ketogenic system will kick in, providing alternative fuel for your body.

Instead of refined carbohydrates made from white flour and white sugar, try to find whole grains with a high fiber content and eat a variety of healthy fats. The ketogenic diet (or "keto" diet) is another potential option for reducing harmful bacteria in the body. Although it is not a good option for everyone, the keto diet, even on a temporary basis, can assist the body in defeating harmful bacteria.

Although fat has been vilified in our culture, good fats are actually highly necessary to your body's essential functioning, especially in the brain and gut. For the last few decades, sugar has been used as a cheaper alternative to fat, which has been falsely accused of making us fat. Sugar, especially in the astronomical amounts it is added into modern foods, is a much more harmful substance than fat. "Low fat" foods are pumped full of sugar to make them palatable, as fat is the ingredient in foods that make them taste good. Fats also help us feel full faster. A high-fat diet is essential to mental, emotional, and physical health. If you do nothing else for your wellbeing, add healthy fats! Even dairy fats such as butter, cream, and whole milk are healthier than you think, especially if they are organically sourced.

Some people gain a lot of benefits from "paleo," "whole foods," or other holistic-type diets. Work with a nutritionist and find what works best with your own health, needs, and lifestyle; however, if you want to change your life, you have got to change your diet.

Even slightly lowering processed carbs and emphasizing healthy fats, proteins, and raw whole vegetables and fruits can make a difference, though. If a highly strict diet will be too much for you to stick with at first, start by making changes you can stick to, and then do it.

In fact, I recommend keto diets as temporary "resets," rather than as long-term solutions. Carbs are necessary to the human diet and keto diets are safer if used on a meaningful temporary basis. Work with a nutritionist to find the best diet plan for you.

No matter what diet plan you use, you must balance your gut biome with probiotics, prebiotics, and polyphenols. These food substances assist beneficial bacteria in the gut, which are essential to vitality.

You might also wish to research cleanses that are designed to eliminate harmful bacteria in the gut. Again, use these with competent advice and be aware that some people experience "die off" reactions; however, decreasing bad bacteria and increasing good bacteria is the most important thing you can do in improving your overall wellness.

Importantly, bacterial balance is directly tied to mental and emotional wellness. Our thoughts, beliefs, and habits contribute to our vitality (or lack thereof).

If you believe that the end of life begins at 30 and it's "all downhill" from there, you will likely have strong emotional responses to everything that seems to "prove" that you are aging. You might run one mile and wake up stiff and sore the next day, then accept that as concrete proof that you are done for, physically speaking. You might then spend precious time berating yourself, eating carbs to make yourself feel better, and engaging in other negative behaviors to try and compensate.

By contrast, if you believe that any person of any age has many good years ahead of them, physical examples of aging will roll off, hardly affecting you at all. You might run one mile and wake up grateful for the soreness that proves you can still run a mile – something that many people in this world are not even capable of, due to physical disabilities that make it impossible. You will then spend time planning how to be less sore the next time you run that mile (or even further).

When you entertain negative beliefs you block yourself mentally, emotionally, and physically. Your stress levels increase and your hormones change, further blocking your potential.

Stress hormones are directly related to accelerated aging. Cortisol, the stress hormone, is responsible for declining health in mid-life.

The human body was not designed for the civilized live of the past century or so. Pre-modern life involved stress, of course, but it was acute stress; that is, people experienced danger or turmoil in brief, separated episodes. Their bodies secreted cortisol to signal that they were endangered. They took those signals to flee or fight or change their circumstances, after which their cortisol levels returned to normal.

Recently, however, humans experience low-level stress almost 100% of the time. With no time to recover, the adrenal system (which manages cortisol) quickly gets depleted. Depleted adrenals create further imbalances throughout the body, like a chain reaction.

Anything that stresses the body triggers the release of cortisol, including, but not limited to, injury, illness, financial difficulties, poor diet, drugs and medications, technology use, social comparison, extreme dieting, pressure at work, arguments, conflict, and a variety of other common human experiences. Because we are hyper-aware of the global strife that plagues our world today, we are almost never not stressed. Eating on the go is another modern stressor that used to be rare but is now the norm.

Under normal circumstances, the human body does such a wonderful job at regulating stress that your adrenaline levels naturally spike at a conflict and then return to normal once the threat has passed. However, most of us today live lives of constant pressure: at work, at home, in our neighborhoods, with our families, everywhere. People today even joke about having to recover from our vacations! Modern life can be summed up with three words: go, go, go. We rarely take the time we need to recuperate and rest, and our bodies are telling the tale.

Further, you do not actually have to be in a situation of stress to experience stress – even remembering the stress is enough to trigger flight or fight more. For example, if you are spending hours lying awake at night worrying about something, it is cortisol that actually keeps you awake. You obviously cannot solve the problem while lying in bed, and the problem is not actually right in front of you at that moment, but your body reacts as if it is. Your body cannot distinguish between the hormones that kept our ancestors safe from a saber tooth tiger attack and the stress of a promotion at work.

As you develop healthy physical habits, you must also develop healthy mental and emotional habits. If you continue to dwell in negative belief patterns, your body will not be able to function at its optimal level. You can literally think yourself sick by stressing, as your hormones secrete adrenaline and leave you unbalanced.

Of course, you cannot control your circumstances, but vitality means learning to approach them from a place of balance and serenity. Vitality means operating at your best mental, emotional, spiritual and physical levels. Vitality is the difference between thriving and merely surviving.

Unfortunately, much of humanity today operates under survival mode. Even in a world with an abundance of wealth and opportunity, we still drag ourselves around in a haze of fear and discomfort. Although Western society has developed a variety of laborsaving and lifesaving devices, it has failed us in many ways. To survive, we develop unhealthy coping mechanisms that further undermine our health and wellbeing.

To regain vitality, we must adjust all dimensions of our being: mental (thought patterns), emotional (traumas, worries, and fears), spiritual (true selves), and physical (diet and exercise). By combining food, rest, sleep, exercise, and other physical changes with the underlying mental, emotional, and spiritual needs, we can essentially "reverse" the aging process and find ourselves healthier and happier than before.

Many of us work in restrictive environments or live in chaotic, stressful places. The stress of making a living, maintaining a social life, and keeping up our health feels like it takes too much out of us, leaving us no time to really *live*.

We were not born to pay bills and then die. We were born with talents, gifts, skills, dreams, visions, goals, and all other kinds of meaningful life purposes. Some of us are gifted artists or dancers or musicians, others are helpers or builders or organizers; we all have different abilities, but many of us have buried (or been buried) ourselves beneath the struggle to survive. We have buried ourselves so deep that we no longer remember what it is to thrive.

Any plan to increase your wellbeing must include a stress reduction component. Of course, working out itself will flood your body with oxytocin, the happiness hormone; the simple act of moving can release tension in your tissues. However, merely working out is not enough. The flight or fight response literally stores tension in our tissues as we literally and metaphorically "freeze" at signs of stress.

When you face imminent danger (like our ancestors faced wild animal attacks), your breath becomes ragged while you are dealing with the threat; it returns to normal when the threat passes. When we face chronic, low-level stress, however, your breath might never return to normal. We face daily stressors that leave our bodies breathless, tense, and "frozen" from fear. It takes a toll.

Pay attention to your neck and shoulders right now. Are you holding them stiff? Or are they loose and relaxed? What about your jaw? Your back? Take regular time to check in with your muscles and release any tension in them and begin a plan today to release old tensions and stresses. Since we literally store trauma in our bodies, it is imperative to let it loose. There are trauma release exercises you can do on your own, or you can find a bodywork specialist to help with this process. Deep tissue massages, Reiki, yoga, and other stress-relieving treatments work wonders on this as well, especially if you go in with the intention to release stress and keep it off.

Keeping our bodies free of unneeded stress and tension goes a long way to maintaining our vitality. Due to the constant stress in our lives many of us are chronic shallow breathers and that deprives our organs, tissues, and cells of vital oxygen on a continuous basis and we don't even notice it. Conscious breathing exercises help with returning our bodies to their optimum states.

If you observe a newborn breathing, you will see the his or her lower belly gently rising and falling in an easy, rhythmic motion. If you watch most adults breathe, however, you will notice most of the movement comes from the upper chest with obvious and exaggerated movement in an attempt to receive enough air. Shallow, inefficient breathing is a serious issue in modern humans, who have forgotten mindful ways of breathing. If you watch a yoga teacher, singer, or accomplished meditator breathe, you will find the pattern much more like the newborn's way of breathing.

Shallow breathing is a learned habit from the many times you froze up during a fight or flight situation. As we collect traumas over time, our breathing gets shallower and shallower, and we develop health issues and hold on to even more traumas as a result.

That is why healing from trauma is hard: we stored that trauma initially in an effort not to feel it. Once it builds up, it gets more difficult to let go of. However, the only way out is through – learning to release old trauma can help you deal with traumas in the future. In the same way that you got used to living with less oxygen, you can acclimatize yourself to more. As a result, you will gain strength, energy, and resilience, perhaps more than you have ever had before.

Without proper air, your body is limited in *all* of its functions, including sleep, digestion, movement, and others. To keep your body strong, healthy, and free of trauma, practice regular conscious breathing until it becomes unconscious. Just 5-10 minutes of mindful breathing every day will go a long way, even if it's just singing in the shower or in the car. The more you re-train yourself to breathe naturally, the more your body will heal itself, with very little effort on your part.

Research methods like the Wim Hof Method, Buteyko Breathing, yogic breathing, and other breathing exercises that suit you best. There are dozens of apps, YouTube videos, books, programs, and other resources that can help you return to the natural breathing you used as a baby. Deep breathing will oxygenate your body and your stress will melt away.

You can combine deep breathing with an Epsom salt bath, essential oils, herbal remedies, or other stress reducing techniques. Research them yourself or find a competent practitioner to guide you, but some common stress-reducing herbs include lavender, chamomile, peppermint, or lemon balm. Indian ayurvedic herbs, such as Ashwaganda and holy basil, are also good options. These are only a few examples of the many resources you can use – try a few and see what works best for you.

Herbs can be taken as supplements, drunk as teas, diffused, or rubbed on as essential oils, added to lotions or laundry, sprayed on pillows and sheets, or used in a variety of other creative and helpful ways. If you have nothing else on hand, time spent dancing or listening to music can work wonders.

By combining these principles and techniques, you can transform from a state of automatic surviving to automatic thriving. Your "default mode" can grow into vitality, no matter your stage of life.

CHAPTER 3

TAMING THE MIND

The cliché about how "if you love your job, you will never work a day in your life" applies to fitness. We are taught that working out has to be painful, through sayings like, "no pain, no gain," and "you get out what you put in."

While these sayings might be true, to a point, sometimes we take them too far. We mangle our bodies through strict workout regimens, and we punish ourselves if we miss even once. We give ourselves difficult diets and then binge on sugar when we fail. We set ourselves up for failure and then when we ultimately fail we blame ourselves, rather than the systems that put us there in the first place.

These patterns come from our subconscious programming, which comes from what we are taught by society, family, and friends.

Remember when you read that willpower is a replenishable resource, like a muscle? Well, just because it can be developed does not mean that it's easy. In many ways, your mind is the hardest muscle to work. That's because it does not function on the physical level. Your mind is working at lightning speed, 100% of the time. Even while you sleep, your brain is working. That's a good thing, by the way.

However, your brain is a powerhouse of conscious and subconscious thoughts, and they tell your body how to function, what to do, where to go, who to be, and literally every other thing you need to keep yourself going.

You literally create your own reality through the programing of your subconscious mind. Your subconscious mind is much more powerful than you think.

The reason that willpower is so hard to develop is because it often has to go against the grain of decades of subconscious training. You have been thinking similar thoughts most of your life, mostly likely, so the minute you try to change them, you run up against resistance.

That's why new habits are so hard to form, and so easy to break. We all know that most New Year's resolutions are broken by February. That's because people usually start by using willpower, instead of mindfulness.

Your subconscious mind is much, much bigger than your conscious mind. Have you ever driven or walked somewhere, only to arrive and realize you don't remember a single part of the trip? That's because subconscious thinking got you there. The subconscious mind is a powerful thing, and it is creating your reality every single minute of every single day.

The trouble is that the subconscious mind is like a pool of water. It's deep, still, and powerful, but it's also easy to move. Little ripples of information are constantly filtering through your subconscious mind, and the ripples are not always correct.

For instance, if you live in Western culture today, you probably have deeply programed beliefs about what it means to be fit, attractive, beautiful, whatever. Your entire life you have been fed magazine images, social media posts, advertisements, sayings, medical information, dietary guidelines, and other information about what it means to be healthy and desirable. No matter how much you tell yourself in the mirror that you are beautiful just the way you are, you look at yourself and still probably think, "fat."

Unless you deliberately re-program your subconscious mind, you will struggle to change your conscious reality. If you have ever bravely set out on a new diet or exercise plan, lost quite a bit of weight, and then ended up right back where you started (or worse), your subconscious mind probably played a role.

In fact, your subconscious mind may have sabotaged your efforts. It is trying to stay stable and safe. Your conscious mind is the one that wants to grow and change; your subconscious mind is just repeating the patterns it has learned its whole life.

Almost like a computer, your subconscious is running "programs" you have downloaded from society, your family, your friends, and yourself.

The good news is, though, is that you are not a computer. You can take out the program and put in a new one at will. It will take dedication, but it is necessary and worth it.

Willpower is what helps us overcome subconscious programming, but it needs to be used mindfully and deliberately. Willpower, like a muscle, gets tired.

If you spent all day, every day in a gym, never stopping to rest or stretch, your muscles would eventually give out. You would probably injure yourself and spend months in recovery. Then you would be back to square one with your exercise routine.

In the same way, willpower can be depleted if you try to attempt making your life changes through sheer force of will. Have you ever seen a bird flying in a storm? Birds instinctively know to fly *with* the wind, rather than against it. In the rare occasions that they do fly directly into the wind, they tire very easily and don't get very far. By using wind currents to move themselves mindfully in the direction they want to go, they get much further, much faster.

You can do the same. Instead of jumping face-first into another new diet or exercise plan, why not take a look at the conscious programming that keeps you in the same patterns you have been in your whole life?

Earlier, you wrote down some of your beliefs about your body image, your weight, and other fitness beliefs. Being aware is a powerful and necessary step.

However, simply being aware is not enough.

You will need to work diligently, today and every day, to re-frame the way you think and feel about yourself on every level, all the way down to your subconscious.

If you have ever heard about manifesting, also called the Law of Attraction, you know that it is a system that allows people to re-program their subconscious mind to draw whatever they want to them effortlessly and easily.

The Law of Attraction is a powerful tool, and of course you are welcome to use it, but many people forget that the Law of Attraction has two parts: thoughts and inspired actions.

It is the *actions* that people so often leave out. By using mindful actions, you can make immediate and powerful shifts in the way you do literally everything in your life.

Instead of working out because you "have to," or because you are afraid of gaining weight, try working out because it is something you love and you want to give yourself the permission to take care of yourself. Instead of punishing yourself for days when you don't work out or eat something you feel you shouldn't, why not grant yourself the kindness of understanding why you are making that choice in the first place?

The trouble is, many of us work out or diet because we feel we "have" to, and we do it in ways that are not necessarily good for us. Everyone is different, and what one person loves another person might be literally incapable of doing safely. Your own individual needs are more important than any arbitrary standard of what it means to be fit.

That being said, you can re-frame your subconscious beliefs to work *for* you, rather than against you. By mindfully questioning your thought processes, you can get to the heart of the issue and bypass all that subconscious programming that is weighing you down.

That way, everything you do is a conscious decision. Even if you *do* decide to skip leg day, you are making that choice from a place of heart-centered thought, instead of yelling at yourself for doing so. When you mindfully weigh your decisions from a place of compassion for yourself, you make those decisions from a place of groundedness.

The next time you are anguishing over whether or not to work out or to eat that slice of cake, ask yourself some questions:

What would I choose to do regarding this thing or issue if I really, truly loved and appreciated myself?

_____

_____

_____

_____

_____

_____

_____

_____

What would I choose if my wellbeing came first and if I really mattered?

_____

_____

_____

_____

_____

_____

_____

What would I choose now if I were not ruled by my unhealed, hurt, unconscious parts of me?

_____

_____

_____

_____

_____

_____

_____

_____

Asking these questions will bring your decision into your conscious mind, rather than your subconscious mind. If you do make the decision not to work out or to still eat the cake, you will be doing it from a place of authority. You have become your own master – that is willpower.

However, the more you practice this, the more you will find yourself realizing that your subconscious programming was merely trying to sabotage you.

Your subconscious mind says things like, "you're too lazy to work out," and "of course you want to eat that, fatty."

Your subconscious mind is built on generations of negative, toxic beliefs about weight, health, fitness, womanhood, money, and all kinds of complicated dimensions. Teasing out where these beliefs come from help you "catch" them in the act, and, more often than not, re-route your mind before it gets too far.

As you practice mindfulness regarding your workout needs and habits, start to notice the kinds of foods, activities, times, people, clothing, and other circumstances that help you want to take care of yourself better. If you notice that you tend to skip your workouts on Saturdays, that tells you something. Plan your week in such a way that you will enjoy your time taking care of yourself and circumnavigate subconscious programming before it even starts.

The more you develop a mindful attitude toward working out, the stronger your willpower will get. As you make conscious choices to do this or that, your willpower will grow until you have to have the conversation with yourself much less often.

You will even start to enjoy your fitness routine, because you will have tailored it to your own needs.

As you do so, ask yourself some more questions and jot down your answers:

Why do you want to lose weight? Do you think others will accept, admire, or like you more, or maybe even be jealous of you if your body will be in top shape? Do you want that to happen? How much importance do you give to how others think about you and your looks? Do you feel like a failure if you do not meet a certain standard? How do you feel about other women who seem to look better than you?

If you are being honest with yourself, questions can be summed up with one word: fear.

We are all afraid of things—being alone, being unwanted, being unhealthy, being rejected by others, being a failure...I can go on, but you get the point.

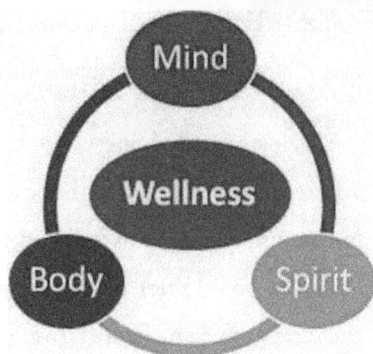

The truth is, fear will never motivate you enough. Fear motivates in the short term, of course, but long-term fear is devastating and unhealthy. As we discussed in a previous chapter, chronic anxiety, stress, and worry leads to serious health consequences. Fear is the same.

Everyone has the right to be loved, supported, respected, and cherished by others around them. Some of us have romantic partners or family members, some prefer friendships, and many of us have some combination of both. It is natural and normal for you want to look your best and fit in with those around you. It's part of our biological evolution.

However, if your motivation to stay fit is out of fear that you will not measure up to *anyone* else's expectations (yes, anyone's), you will fail. Fear is simply not a good motivator, long-term.

Fear is not a good motivator because it is external. External motivation is much less effective than internal motivation, also called intrinsic motivation.

Even if you believe you are seeking fitness for yourself, you will want to be very, very honest with yourself about where your fitness goals come from. If you are consistently doing well and making progress over years of steady, concerted effort, the chances are good that you are intrinsically motivated. If not, your motivation probably comes from elsewhere.

Being brutally honest about where your motivation comes from (inside yourself, or elsewhere) might be a painful conversation to have with yourself, but it is necessary. You will continue to find yourself right back where you started if you do not re-frame your subconscious programming and decide that you want to be fit and strong for *you* – no one else.

Make a commitment to yourself: you are the source of your motivation.

Once you have made that commitment, you will be able to motivate yourself more easily, more often. Soon, you will be finding it hard to do things that were easy before and easy to do things that seemed impossible, even a short while ago.

Be patient with yourself, however. Remember, you have years of subconscious programming to overcome, and it is trying to tell you to keep your motivations outside of yourself.

Your subconscious mind is a *passive* brain function; your conscious mind is an *active* one. Choosing to be the author of your own story means taking ownership of your own thoughts and actions, rather than leaving them up to Fate or your mother or the way someone looked at you today in the grocery store.

To discover where you are on that path, you can ask yourself a difficult and life-altering question: *Am I the heroine of my life or am I a victim of my circumstances? Do I want to be the heroine or victim of my life?*

As you work through some of these things, you might want to find a way to keep yourself accountable. Finding an accountability partner on a similar journey might help, as will finding a fitness coach or trainer you trust to allow you to find your own way. Finding a gym or club or other group of like-minded people can be helpful as well, even if it's an online "tribe" of people into the same fitness goals as you are.

Only you know for sure what works best for you, so try out a few things and see what works. Do not hesitate to make a change if it's not working out, but make sure you stick with it long enough to be sure. As you make more mindful choices, you will be more aware of your decision-making process and what plans and programs work for you.

MANAGING EMOTIONS

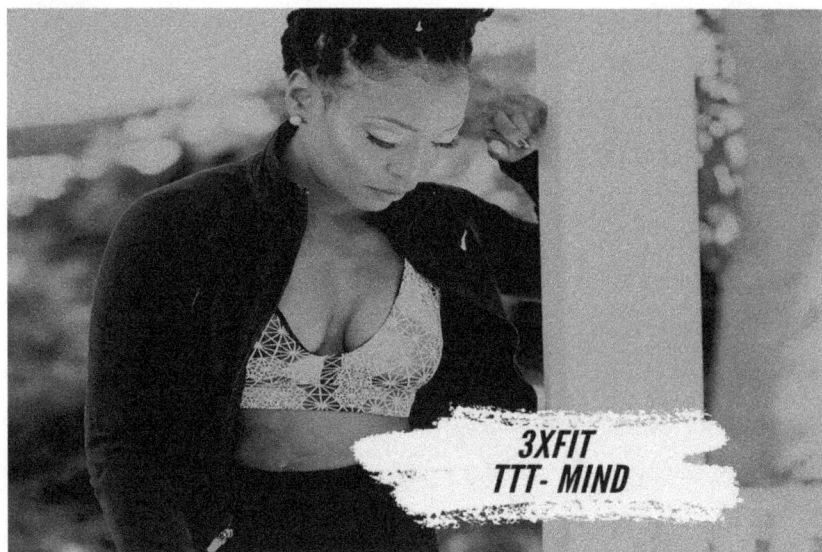

As I mentioned previously, emotions left unprocessed get trapped in your body as trauma. Your mental and emotional processes go hand in hand, as you have been taught since the day of your birth the "right" ways to express emotion.

We are also taught what kinds of emotions are appropriate to express—mainly positive ones, as it turns out.

However, we all know that negative emotions crop up eventually, whether we like it or not. When we choke them back or let them explode all over the place, they can get "frozen" in our cells as trauma. Expressing our emotions in a balanced and healthy way is key to overall wellness and clarity.

The truth is that there are no "good" emotions and "bad" emotions. There are just emotions, and they are here to help us.

Emotions are signals of how our body is feeling. Emotions provide clues to what we need to keep us functioning optimally. Often, emotions give clearer direction than our thoughts, if we listen to them carefully and without judgment.

Unfortunately, we are also taught that feeling "good" is selfish and wrong, even while we are not allowed to express anger or sorrow or any of the so-called "bad" emotions. It's a contradiction we all face.

When you were born, your survival literally depended on expressing emotions. When you smiled, you were praised. When you cried, you were given treats and toys to calm you down and stop you crying.

Although these were natural and inevitable responses designed to help you communicate before you could talk, the residual effects are still with us.

Due to the ways we were taken care of as infants and the ways we were taught growing up to express ourselves (or not to express ourselves, as the case may be), trapped emotions in the body are common.

You probably have emotions trapped in your cells, which can rise to the surface whenever you begin to change your lifestyle. When your body starts to "wake up," these emotions "shake loose." This is a good thing – your body is trying to let go of what no longer serves it. However, it might be uncomfortable for you if you are suddenly more emotional than usual, especially if you still have subconscious programming that teaches you that emotions are inappropriate.

A mindful approach to emotions can help. If, when you begin your new quest for vitality and fitness, you suddenly find yourself irritable, sad for "no reason," or prone to random fits of joy, observe these emotions, thank them, and let them go. They are releasing themselves, and it's a good thing.

Keep at it, even if it gets to be overwhelming. Be gentle to yourself and seek help from a trusted friend or professional if you need it. Venting can work wonders for trapped emotions, as can therapeutic treatments such as massage or yoga, or more intense forms of release like kickboxing or running. Some people scream into pillows or deliberately break or throw things in safe, controlled environments to get out extra feelings.

Do what is best for you and seek support as needed. Trust the process and know that the more emotions you can release, the more your body will be able to process future emotions safely.

Over time, your body will lean into its new pattern of processing emotions and thoughts in mindful, meaningful ways. You will grow more balanced, centered, and healthy in every possible way. You might also lose weight naturally, without even trying! Sometimes, that's all the body needs.

In fact, you might find yourself feeling happier and calmer more often, and "for no reason." Instead of feeling upset "for no reason" (which is actually your body signaling that you are running negative subconscious programming), you will begin to naturally feel good, without even trying. Less coping with food, more simple joy.

CHAPTER 4

RECALIBRATE YOUR BODY
FOR OPTIMUM PERFORMANCE

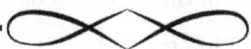

I n modern, Western society, with our poor diets, lack of movement, negative beliefs about health and wellness, constant stress, and a whole host of other problems, women get the short end of the stick.

Hormonal imbalances that play a role in menstrual cycles, perimenopause, and menopause are further challenges to overcome. No wonder women over 40 are among the least happy!

THE HORMONAL COCKTAIL

Menopause is a crucial time in the life of any woman. During menopause, our bodies change on the hormonal level as we switch from one phase of life to the next. Your hormones regulate the most crucial systems in your body and need to be functioning at the optimum level in order to keep everything running effectively. Unfortunately, during menopause your hormones are already fluctuating, so it is even easier to get thrown off track.

Menopause includes a variety factors that further affect weight loss, including hormonal fluctuations, loss of muscle mass due to the aging process, reduced physical activity, inadequate sleep, and high insulin resistance that makes it more difficult to lose weight. Further, the symptoms of menopause (including hot flashes, a slowed metabolism, and other changes) make it more difficult to stay diligent with exercise and eating routines.

Women during menopausal changes often gain weight rapidly due to these significant changes in all body systems. Muscle mass starts to decrease and body fat increases, both in the subcutaneous fat just below the skin and in the fatty tissues deeper within the body.

Subcutaneous fat just below the skin is the fat that worries us about our looks, but it is the visceral fat (deep in our tissues) that is a greater cause for concern. Visceral fat leads to health problems such as difficulty breathing, cholesterol problems, high blood pressure, Type 2 diabetes, heart disease, and other weight-related issues.

Thus, it's clear that maintaining a healthy weight in menopause is not merely about our appearance and self-esteem. It's important to maintain our vitality to slow the aging process and make sure our mid-life years are our best years. Your later years will be improved, too.

The good news is that you can keep your hormones in balance by following the tips and principles in this book. This section focuses on how to understand the underlying processes of menopause in terms of your health and fitness goals to give you a "leg up" on overcoming them.

Your most important hormone is oxytocin, the "feel good" hormone. You release oxytocin during pleasurable experiences, such as looking a cute dog or eating your favorite food.

Next on our list is cortisol, the stress hormone. You release cortisol under stress, which can lead to all kinds of issues which we have previously discussed. The most important part for this section, though, is that cortisol represses your ability to burn fat. You must be relaxed to make any progress.

After cortisol is insulin, which regulates blood sugar. I discuss sugar in a later chapter, but for now it is enough to know that if your diet is overwhelmed with carbohydrates and sugar, your insulin will be out of whack.

These next hormones are the most crucial during perimenopause and menopause: estrogen, progesterone, and testosterone. These hormones are influenced by oxytocin, cortisol, and insulin, and are already experiencing changes during this time of life.

Hormonal shifts lead to increased insulin resistance, meaning that your cells do not effectively absorb and utilize the insulin your body secretes. Increased insulin resistance increases your risk for heart troubles, cancer, memory function, and other serious effects.

Changes in your estrogen levels naturally lead to weight gain, as estrogen affects several crucial body systems. When estrogen levels decrease in menopause, the body must adjust accordingly. Weight gain often follows, although estrogen decrease is not directly responsible for the change.

Estrogen controls cholesterol levels, maintains bone health, and regulates the menstrual cycle. As these systems shift in menopause, your metabolism drops, as well. These changes lead to excess body fat as your habits and body systems struggle to keep up with the changes.

Further, both progesterone and estrogen affect how your cells respond to insulin. Your blood sugar levels are tied to the way your body produces insulin, which is tied to your hormone production. Shifts in the way your body handles sugar means that maintaining or losing weight is more difficult.

Not only do the hormones regulate sugar processing, they also regulate the way your body handles stress. Your sex hormones (estrogen, progesterone, and testosterone) regulate your monthly cycle and must be in balance for optimum health. Cortisol, however, changes your production of these hormones because they are related to your reproductive system.

Cortisol signals the body that it is not time to procreate—it's time to be afraid. Once cortisol overwhelms the system, all other hormones are thrown out of balance.

Weight loss is more effective when you are not stressed. Stress causes the body to keep and gain weight, as the body is attempting to store fat to keep you going in a crisis. Like a camel storing water for the dry spell of crossing the desert, stress signals your body to save all it can for a time when there is no food available.

However, you likely have plenty of food available, so the extra fat is not necessary. In fact, it is dangerous in large quantities. Letting your body know that it is safe to lose weight is crucial by reducing your stress, including a healthier diet. Unhealthy diets are significant stressors on the body, on top of all the other stressors discussed throughout this book.

To recalibrate your body and allow your hormones to rebalance themselves, you will have to make changes to the ways you eat and exercise. Increasing feel-good hormones and decreasing cortisol will make an impact in your overall health and wellbeing. As you balance your hormones, your body systems will come back online.

A variety of alternative and complementary therapies have been shown to be effective tools to help with balancing hormones, especially during menopause and perimenopause. Following the guidelines in this book will be helpful, especially alongside other tools such as yoga, hypnosis, meditation, herbal remedies, psychotherapy, acupuncture, and more. Explore options that work for you and incorporate a wide variety of assistance to your regimen. Your body, mind, and spirit will thank you!

YOUR FOOD SHOULD BE YOUR MEDICINE

As previously discussed, filling your diet with as much organic, free-range, pasture-raised, pesticide free, hormone free, and otherwise clean foods as possible will turn your life around. Redefining what counts as "healthy" and thinking of your food as medicine is a big step, but it's worth it.

When you eat junk food and then try to combat the results after the fact, you make very little progress. When you think of food as medicine and prevent problems before they arise, you are already ahead of the game.

Reducing the toxic load of our food is crucial because toxins hinder the body's ability to keep itself toxin-free. Your body has natural detox systems in place, but these can get quickly overloaded, especially if you are stressed.

First, you need to decrease the amount of toxins you take in, then use supportive foods to help your body detox.

Unfortunately, toxins are now ubiquitous, even in things like tap water. Tap water is filled with fluoride, which is supposed to be good for you but is way overused, and it also is filled with artificial hormones, excess antibiotics, and other chemicals from our water system. Bottled water is sometimes literally just tap water put in a plastic bottle, so be cautious. Try to avoid tap water as much as you can, and consider filtering the water you use for drinking, cooking, and bathing.

Another significant toxin in our food is monosodium glutamate (MSG). Salt is another food that has been vilified but is actually a necessary nutrient, but the real trouble is that the salt we eat today is highly processed and therefore dangerous. High quality sea salt, Himalayan salt, or other naturally derived salts are much safer for the body and provide essential nutrients if used in healthy doses.

Saturated fats and trans-fats (such as vegetable oils, canola oil, and other processed oils) are not only harmful, they are in most foods. Replacing your current fat intake with healthier fats such as avocado oil, coconut oil, organic butter, ghee, and other healthy fats will prevent your body from working overtime just to handle dangerous forms of fat.

As mentioned above, your gut biome is key to your health. Fermented foods such as yogurt, kefir, sauerkraut, miso, kimchi, and other naturally preserved foods contain beneficial bacteria that feed your gut biome. Wherever possible, make these foods yourself or buy them from less-processed sources—processing affects the strains of bacteria and can lessen their effects.

Important prebiotics (which feed probiotics) include chicory root, Jerusalem artichoke, dandelion leaves, garlic, onions, leeks, asparagus, bananas, barley, oats, apples, cocoa, flaxseed, wheat bran, and seaweed. These foods also assist the body in detoxing itself.

By lessening your toxin intake and regularly detoxing, you can increase your vitality by allowing your body to function at the optimum level.

A NOTE ON DETOXING

Your body uses a compound called glutathione as a cleanser for your liver, kidneys, lymphatic system, and other detoxification systems. Our liver, in particular, is filled with glutathione, which is naturally produced by the body to clean out anything that does not suit us. However, aging, alcohol intake, stress, and other factors reduce the amount of glutathione, causing issues throughout the body.

Certain vegetables such as broccoli, kale, cabbage, cauliflower, and Brussels sprouts contain glutathione in abundance. Eating detox foods such as cruciferous greens will assist your body in cleansing itself. Good fats, too, assist your body in processing these foods optimally.

Herbal teas and green teas can be highly cleansing, and there are a variety of detox teas available to suit your own needs and tastes. Lemon, ginger, holy basil (tulsi), and rooibos teas are good choices. Detox products like activated charcoal or diatomaceous earth can also help – make sure you get plenty of extra water when you use them, however.

Minerals in the body assist with detoxing, so you should make sure you are getting enough. The earth's water and soil are depleted of the essential minerals we need to thrive, so adding minerals to your diet is always a good option. Supplement with mineral tablets or find vitamins that include minerals to ensure your body has an adequate supply. If you have the opportunity to go to a mineral spa and soak in a mineral tub or spring, do it! Absorbing minerals through your skin is the most effective, so try Epsom salt baths or mineral sprays or lotions if a mineral spa is not accessible to you. Bone broth is another powerful source of digestive cleansing and is filled with minerals and nutrients that assist your body with cleansing.

Taking a "liquid fast" from time to time by drinking only soups, smoothies, broths, teas, and other nutritious drinks for a 24-hour period can also assist your body in resetting itself and purging anything it no longer needs. Fasting allows the body to "catch up" with the strenuous labor of digesting by letting any old food matter to work itself through your digestive system.

Some people who fast choose to go without all food and water for 2-3 meals as a similar option, although once a month is plenty for this option. Going without food should be a choice you make to reset your body, not a way to deprive yourself of essential nutrients and calories in an attempt to lose weight. Healthy fasting means returning to gently to an adequate diet once you have finished your fast, without gorging yourself or trying to see how long you can go.

Ketogenic diets and intermittent fasting can also assist the body in moving toxins out naturally, although you should research and meet with a competent nutritionist to decide what is best for you and your health needs. Many women have also found that getting plenty of proteins and dairy strengthens their muscles and bones, as well as getting plenty of soluble fiber to keep their digestives systems clean and regular. Foods such as broccoli, avocados, Brussel sprouts, and flaxseeds contain plenty of fiber and will help your body regulate itself.

Many people experience a "detox reaction" whenever they undergo a new diet or fast. This is normal, and you should allow your body the kindness it needs during this time. You might see an increase of symptoms or a need for more sleep; you might also notice emotional fluctuations or mood swings. This is okay – your body is losing what no longer serves it and will come back better than before.

By decreasing your sugar, white flour, and processed food intake and increasing your intake of whole grains, vegetables, fruits, and other wholesome foods, you will allow your body to naturally overcome the challenges of menopause by giving it the fuel it needs to thrive.

Also, menopause means that your body can actually get by on less food than you ate in your 20s and 30s. By decreasing the number of calories you take in on a daily basis, you can allow your body to process the food you take in more efficiently.

However, this does not mean that you skimp on nutrients. Quality is more important than quantity, and it is crucial that you increase your vitamin and nutrient intake through your food.

In fact, many women find a vegetarian or vegan diet to be a good choice for them in this time of life. Plant matter is a powerhouse of nutrient-dense goodness, and plant-based diets allow the avoidance of excess hormones and additives in a variety of meat products.

Vegetables and fruits are superfoods. They are life-giving storehouses of micronutrients that have sustained human beings for centuries. Although humans have also always eaten meat, modern meat products contain a variety of added hormones and preservatives and tend to be highly processed. A plant centered diet is healthy for many reasons.

Of course, some choose a vegetarian or vegan lifestyle for religious or social reasons, as consuming meat products can contribute to violence and cruelty around the globe. Vegetarian and vegan diets are more environmentally friendly and allow us to do our part for the planet.

If you do choose to eat meat products, whenever possible, choose grass-fed and organic to decrease the contaminants found in the meat. As always, work with a nutritionist when making significant dietary changes, and take your own health, lifestyle, and other needs into account.

Choosing the correct diet for you must take your health needs into account by making sure you get adequate protein, iron, and other necessary nutrients as part of a full and wholesome diet. Vegetarian and vegan diets can satisfy all your dietary needs but will take some mindful effort in a world that tends to favor eating meat (although that is changing). Plant proteins, dairy, eggs, nuts, and other vegetarian and vegan proteins are powerful sources of nutrients in a plant-based diet. You can have fun being creative about the kinds of nutrients you get in your diet and enjoy the process of nourishing yourself.

Instead of living to eat, eat to live. So much of eating in modern times is about snacking to feel okay again or stuffing our face in the car between appointments. Humans are losing the tendency to eat slowly and mindfully with their loved ones. We eat as a necessity, rather than as a choice.

Eating on the go is actually one of the least healthy things you can do for your body, and yet so many of us do it so many times a day. Eating seems like a guilty pleasure or something we do to keep ourselves alive instead of a necessary part of life.

Even more than that, though, eating is a privilege – so many people on this planet do not have adequate food. In America today, we are blessed with an abundance of food and many varieties of food, and yet we are unable to eat healthfully for all our choices. The great irony is that we have plenty to eat, and yet we are starving ourselves. Even when we overeat, we starve ourselves of essential nutrients that would help allow us to thrive.

Mindfulness in eating can transform your perspective on food and actually increase your nutrient intake. Eating slowly and with gratitude and joy is a simple step you can take to learn to enjoy food for its nourishment and strength.

Your food should be your medicine, first and foremost. The more you make your food your medicine, the less medicine you will ultimately have to take. Since we live in a time filled with choice and variety, learn the choices that are best for you and then stick with them using your newfound perspective and growing willpower.

A nutritious diet is the first step to vitality. Only after balancing your eating can you move on to the next step: moving your body with intelligence.

MOVING YOUR BODY WITH INTELLIGENCE

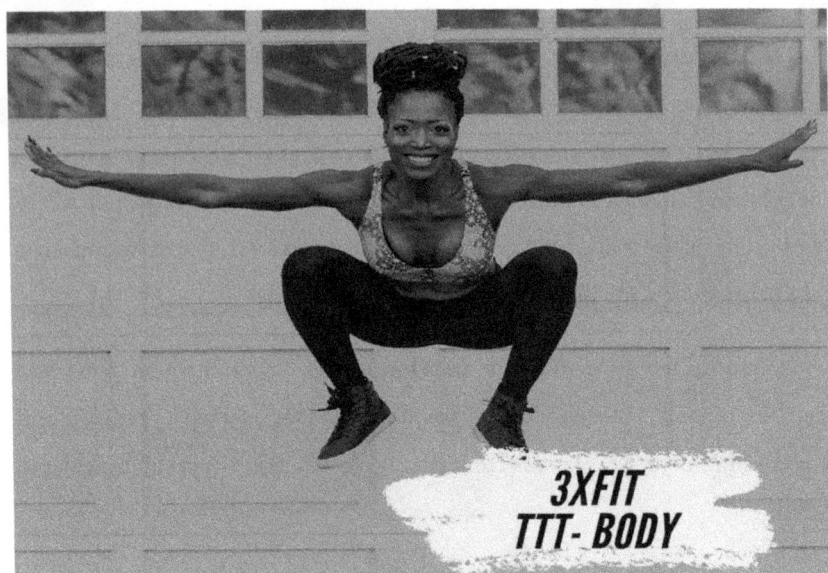

**3XFIT
TTT- BODY**

Western culture values independence, dominance, power, and other hyper-masculine traits. The American ideal of "pulling yourself up by your bootstraps" and "rags to riches" has benefits, certainly, and there is no reason not to try your best. However, we often take these ideals too far. Women especially sometimes need different perspectives to be successful and oftentimes taking the hardcore approach is more harmful than helpful.

Aerobics, for instance, has been a vastly popular form of exercise for a few generations now. The trouble with aerobics, though, is that it requires a head-on approach, and tends to lose its effectiveness over time.

Cardio, in fact, sometimes has an opposite effect. Because it overtaxes the body, it increases stress and actually has an opposite effect. Working out too hard and for too long results in inflammation, soreness, stiffness, and other problems, of course, but it also lessens your body's ability to burn fat.

Other forms of exercise, too, can be overdone if not done intelligently. Hight intensity trainings, weight training, and other anaerobic exercise can be a useful alternative to cardio, but can be taken too far and stress the body too much. Putting too much stress on the body is counterproductive because you ultimately end up where you started.

Menopausal and post-menopausal women, especially, must be careful not to overtax their bodies. When your body goes through hormonal changes, your sex hormones take a step back and allow other systems to take their place, meaning that they can be more easily depleted.

When this happens, your body "goes haywire" trying to keep up with the changes. This results in symptoms like weigh fluctuations, emotional turmoil, and other symptoms.

Stress is the main factor in how effective your workouts are: too much stress actually takes you away from your goals. For instance, cortisol reduces muscle mass in the thighs. As we age, we tend to lose thigh muscle mass, which greatly reduces our mobility into old age. If your cortisol levels are too high, your thighs will decrease over time and you will have issues with recovery and overall strength.

Understanding how hormones, diet, stress, and other factors play a role in weight loss is crucial in making permanent progress that will not require you to train harder and harder to get the same results. Proper exercise, too, will take your focus away from the scale (which is an arbitrary and unreliable measure of health) and place it in more important places, such as muscle mass, toning, and overall wellbeing.

Fat burning is at its peak during anaerobic exercise. Resistance training is a powerful way to base your workout around anaerobic exercise, which is a useful way to lose fat and gain muscle.

Weightlifting, high intensity interval training (HIIT), and other resistance workouts can work wonders, but they can also tire the body and trigger that plateau, so only do resistance workouts every other day or once you have had time to recover from muscle soreness. Instead of increasing the frequency or repetitions, increase the intensity. Your body is wonderfully adaptable and will keep up with you.

Results from resistance training typically plateau in two to three weeks. At that point, you will need to increase the intensity, or your body will stop burning fat.

If you increase the length or frequency of your workouts instead of the intensity, you will hit that plateau. Increasing the length is tempting, since it seems easier to do the same thing for longer, but a few repetitions of heavier weights is actually a more mindful way to look at your workout and will bring you the results you want in the long run.

To avoid plateauing after a few weeks of exercise, use different types of exercise at different times to keep your body from reaching this point. Using both aerobic and anaerobic exercise to keep your body from leveling out will help, so change routines every two to three weeks to keep ahead of yourself. Changing up your routine will also keep your mind engaged in the exercise, which will make it easier to stay motivated and interested, thereby reducing stress even more.

When you do cardio, aim for 65-70% of your heart rate based on your age. Keeping at this optimum level allows your body to function at its best. With cardio, you will need to increase the length of time, rather than the intensity; however, remember quality over quantity. If you are pushing yourself to do hours of running, way past the point of exhaustion, you are actually keeping yourself heavier by forcing your body to store fat instead of release it.

Of course, you will naturally need to invest time and effort into working out. Still, spending all day every day doing low quality, exhausting training actually takes you in the opposite direction of where you want to go. A well-designed resistance training routine with plenty of supplementary exercises built in will take you much further than just trying harder and longer.

No matter the type of exercise you do, you must allow your body time to recover between workouts. It is tempting to think that constant, frenzied effort will help you reach your fitness goals; however, you are likely reading this book because that system has not worked for you. Mindful, deliberate exercise plans that avoid overtaxing the body will actually be more beneficial and will help you meet your fitness goals and keep them. That way, you will not find yourself back in the same place over and over. Allowing at least one day (or more, if need be) between exercises is absolutely essential. Every other day is sufficient.

Meanwhile, you must reduce your stress levels, including stress caused by exercise. If you are constantly stiff, sore, exhausted, and dreading your workouts, you are actually not assisting yourself at all. You are going in the opposite direction from your goal, which is overall wellness and natural, easy weight loss that you can maintain for the rest of your life.

In fact, stress has an optimum level. A small amount of stress stimulates the human growth hormone (HGH), which burns fat and reduces aging as well as growing lean muscle. Intense anaerobic exercise produces HGH and also glucagon, which combats insulin spikes and fuels your cells. Testosterone and adrenaline, too, do their part to help your body release fat and burn it off. Some stress is necessary; too much is detrimental.

CHAIRS ARE THE WORST

There is a scientific debate about whether or not "sitting is the new smoking." Even if it is not as unhealthy as smoking, prolonged sitting is not natural for the body and can have myriad harmful effects.

And Americans, by and large, sit a lot. We sit at work, then we go home and sit in front of the TV, we sit in the car, we sit at restaurants, and pretty much everywhere else. Our day to day lives are filled with very little physical activity, which has a number of harmful effects.

First, it stresses the spine and internal organs. Second, it blocks a number of crucial body systems, including the lymphatic system and circulatory system.

Even more importantly, too much sitting destroys good posture and creates neck, shoulder, and spine problems, as well as unbalanced hips and other structural issues.

If you, like most of us, sit too much, you might run into difficulties when you start a serious exercise program because your body has been used to exerting itself in different ways. You will want to work to correct any imbalances in your spine or posture before you concentrate seriously on an exercise routine. Otherwise, you might injure yourself and set yourself back months or even years.

One option is to go to a chiropractor or other bodywork therapist to assist with straightening your body out. However, another option is a simple one that you can add to your exercise routine: pilates.

Pilates classes and private lessons assist with strengthening your core muscles, which protect your spine, abdomen, lower back, hips and pelvis from injury. Having a strong core benefits all major muscle groups and will make your other workouts even more successful.

If possible, take private pilates lessons to ensure that your instructor can dedicate one-on-one time to correcting any misalignments in your posture. However, group classes can work wonders, as well. If your body is especially prone to misalignment, at least twenty pilates sessions before beginning a serious weight training routine will keep your fitness plans much safer, stronger, and effective. Combining core strength workouts with gentle cardio might be optimum for your level as you first start out.

You might find it beneficial to include a variety of exercise types and formats:

CARDIO

While doing cardio, protect your joints by doing longer, low intensity workouts. The speeds you reached in your 20s and 30s are probably not safe for you, and that is okay. Instead of increasing speed, incline the treadmill and stay on a little longer. However, no need to increase the distance – you can meet your distance goals by taking more time to accomplish them. Cardio workouts can increase oxytocin and even burn some fat if used optimally and without overtaxing the body.

Cardio training tends to support overall weight loss throughout the body, and rarely results in much toning of muscles or shaping of figure.

RESISTANCE TRAINING

To grow muscle mass and tone and shape your body, use a well-designed resistance training program. Weightlifting, strength training machines, and other resistance exercises can keep your body in fat burning mode even hours after you finish exercising, especially if you incorporate intermittent fasting. Resistance training is optimal for fat burning and increases lean muscle and can be an effective stress reducer.

LOW IMPACT ACTIVITIES

Swimming, stretching, dancing, walking, and other low impact activities can be highly beneficial additions to any exercise routine.

If you have back issues, swimming is a good option because if done correctly and with optimum posture, swimming is gentle on the muscles and spine. Backstrokes are particularly safe.

Dancing is another highly beneficial activity, especially because it is engaging. If you are having fun, you are less likely to overstress your body. For that reason, long walks are also recommended.

Of course, stretching is necessary as a warm-up and cool-down from any workout routine, but stretching becomes more and more important as we age due to the way our bodies tend to lose water content and increase in stiffness. At any age, however, holding still too long or limiting our range of motion (such as through sitting or standing at work for long hours) can result in injury if we are not properly warmed up before beginning. From an energetic perspective, stiffness indicates stuck trauma that needs to be dealt with.

If you ever feel too tired, sick, or sore to do your planned exercise for that day, stretch instead. Stretching is highly beneficial and when paired with deep breathing can help detox and de-stress your body and help you recover faster.

CHAPTER 5

THE SPIRIT ASPECTS
OF STAYING FIT & FABULOUS

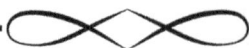

———⟨✕⟩———

How do we distinguish between something "living" and "dead"? When a person dies, it is not because their body leaves. The body is still there. Their spirit, soul, essence, whatever you choose to call it, is the thing that leaves. We distinguish "living" things (trees, animals, plants) from "non-living" things based on their ability to act, think, move, and live on their own.

Your mental, emotional, and physical states are really just components of the main part of you: your spirit.

Dr. Wayne W. Dyer, the "father of motivation," suggested that we are not physical beings having spiritual experiences, we are spiritual beings having physical experiences.

If you look at your life from that perspective, you can realize that your real self is not your physical self that you can see, hear, and touch, but your spiritual self, which goes much further. Your personality, experiences, emotions, and other ephemeral components are the things that make up the essence of you. When we die, the physical part is all that's left, and that is not considered "you," in the end.

To some, the word "spiritual" triggers lots of negative associations. Maybe you have strong objections to the idea of being spiritual, due to the images that flash into your mind when it's mentioned. Perhaps you think of a deeply religious person or an extremely Zen person. Maybe spirituality makes you uncomfortable because you do not believe in a higher power at all. That is okay. You do not need to believe in a higher power, meditate, or attend regular religious meetings to be in tune with your spiritual self.

Simply holding gratitude for the fact that you are alive is a strong start. If you are ill, overweight, and generally miserable, your spirit will feel that energy and keep it going. To be balanced and centered you will want to consider ways of keeping yourself spiritually fit as well as physically fit.

Previously, we discussed about the need for internal, rather than external, motivation. Your spirit is the thing that qualifies you as essentially "alive," but are you really living?

The difference between thriving and surviving is the key to a happy, meaningful life, and it goes hand in hand with health and fitness. A spiritually fulfilled person is a motivated, healthy, balanced person. Vitality is swift to follow.

Spiritual fitness comes in a variety of formats. Some people love meditation or religious practice, others spend time in nature and that's enough. Whatever floats your spiritual boat, however, you will need to make time for it on a daily basis if you want to truly love your life.

A meaningful life includes a key ingredient: meaning. If your life seems purposeless or worthless, finding something to bring meaning will create a 180-degree shift that will influence your health, fitness, and overall wellbeing.

Each of us have different talents, abilities, and purposes that we are born with and acquire throughout our lives. You will not feel fully satisfied with your life until you can, as much as possible, connect with the person you are deep inside.

If you are constantly self-sabotaging yourself, it could be because your true self is not satisfied by your current goals, dreams, and desires. Re-evaluating *why* you want to be fit and strong can go a long way toward understanding how to heal from the inside out.

Personal growth includes regularly evaluating where you are, where you want to go, and how to get there. It does not have to be a massive overhaul each time, nor does it have to be a chore. Finding time to be in tune with your inner self will fill you with the empowerment you need to reach whatever goal you want.

Find ways to check in regularly with your spiritual side. Ask yourself the following questions and jot down your answers:

If you had all the time you needed, what would be your next project or goal? What stresses, anxieties, and obstacles get in the way of your dreams?

_____

_____

_____

_____

_____

_____

_____

Journaling in general is a highly effective tool for understanding your inner self. Keeping a regular record of your thoughts, emotions, actions, and goals will keep you on track, and it will help you understand your life holistically instead of reacting day by day. By viewing your life as a connected whole and tracking your progress you will start to see patterns that can assist you in altering your path.

Vibrancy is not a "one and done" achievement. You will not some day "accomplish" wellness and then never have to deal with it again. If you are putting of doing the things you love because you are waiting until you reach a certain fitness goal, you are going to have a much harder time reaching that goal and keeping it.

Instead, think of your life as many small moments of experience. Some are successes, others are learning opportunities, but all of them connect into the greater whole of you. Even your scars can be decorations if you let them.

Beginning with inner wellness and allowing the outer wellness to follow will allow your inner self to guide the journey, rather than following external waypoints, which might not serve you as well as your internal guide.

As you do this, you might experience pushback from those who are used to seeing you one way. Change is sometimes difficult for people who are accustomed to staying in a rut, but do not let that discourage you. If you trust them, you can explain why you are making these decisions and invite them to join you. After that, the choice is theirs. Only you can decide what is right for you.

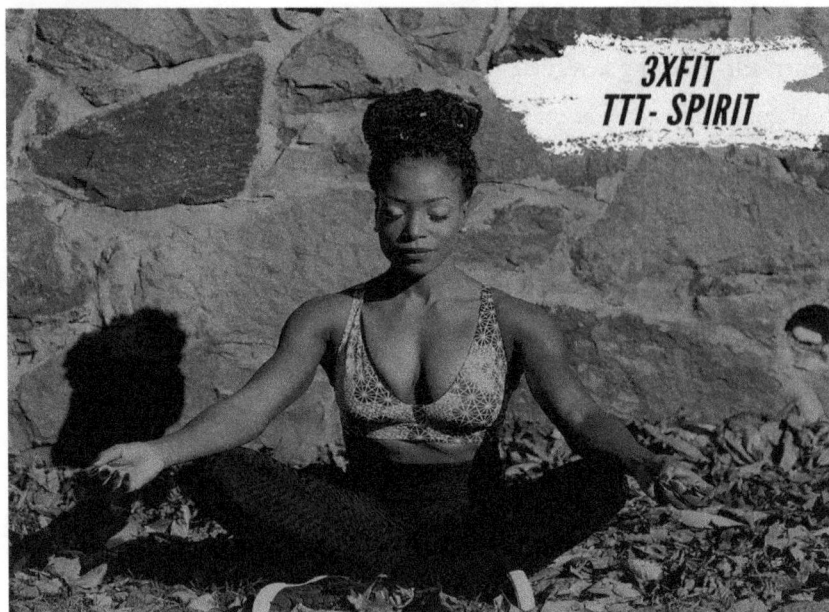

**3XFIT
TTT- SPIRIT**

Some people might drift away. It might be hard, but ultimately the people who stay in your life are the ones that you need the most. In time, new, healthy relationships will replace the ones you leave behind. The old ones will come back when the time is right.

Tuning into your spirituality is not easy, but it is also not complicated.

Another word for the inner knowing of spirituality is intuition. Some people are born with a great deal of intuition, and some have to work harder to develop it. Everyone can develop it if they try, however.

Intuition refers to the "gut vibe" you get when something just feels "off" or intrigues you but you can't figure out why. If you've ever been drawn to a work of art or a pet or a piece of music or anything like that, you know what

I'm talking about. Intuition is an inner knowing that guides and directs us toward people and places and activities and objects that are correct for us.

Often, your intuition speaks from your heart, rather than your head, although not always. Intuition varies from person to person, but everyone has a small inner voice. Growing up, you might have been taught about your "conscience" that keeps you steady on your path. Your intuition recognizes the shared dignity in everyone and will guide you to make higher, healthier choices for yourself and others.

Most importantly, intuition allows you to sense what is right for you in situations so you can start living proactively, rather than reactively. Making intuitive connections between experiences in your life can let you "predict" what will happen in any given situation that comes up. I'm not saying that you will suddenly be able to tell fortunes with a crystal ball; however, you can better inform yourself about anything that happens to you and avoid negative situations and seek positive ones by understanding how each new experience affects you.

In fitness situations, this might look like watching for patterns in your exercise history and choosing trainers, classes, programs, diets, and other tools that are more uniquely suited to your own needs and situation. The more deliberately you navigate your world, the more confidence and power you can gain.

In the end, spirituality is about empowerment. Owning your personal power is the end goal in regaining vitality. It's not about any arbitrary standards of weight or strength; it's about seeing yourself as truly *yourself*— and finding that self to be someone you really love.

Here is a journaling exercise you can do to practice increasing your intuitive gifts. Used alongside regular reflection and maybe even working with a spiritual coach or accountability partner, you can increase your spiritual capacities for lifelong empowerment.

Journaling exercise:

Every single day, write at least three pages in your journal, even if you write "I have nothing to write," over and over. By dumping all of your thoughts, feelings, activities, moods, and other internal processes into your journal you can start to make sense of them and sort them into meaningful categories. Even a bulleted list is fine to start!

How To Conduct Your Transformation

Now that you have explored all dimensions of mind, body, and spirit, you need to create a detailed action plan and then follow through. As you make your plan, focus on what you know you can actually implement, and then do it. There are no valid reasons not to take control of your health and your life. You can do it—you deserve it.

Writing down your plan and working with a fitness coach, mentor, or accountability partner is key. In your planner, block out time for yourself *first*, then fill in the other necessary parts of your day. If you make your fitness a priority, you will be more likely to actually achieve your goals.

As you make your plan, be careful not to overschedule yourself. It is easy to get caught up in the excitement of a new plan and then get into it and realize you are trying to do too much. Keeping your plan realistic from the start is a sure way of making your goals attainable.

Think about how to get your exercise and fitness plans done. Remember, the best plan is one you can stick to, so decide if you want to cook your own meals, cook ahead, or go on a day-by-day basis. Plan according to your own needs and abilities, then stick to it. Using a paper planner is optimal because it cements the reminders in your brain as you hand write them.

If your health plan includes supplements, place them somewhere you won't forget and consider using a pill organizer to keep on track.

Getting up early to give yourself extra time to set your focus for the day and take care of yourself *first* is a crucial step. People tend to be at their most productive in the early hours, before they get bogged down with people and schedules. It is crucial to have some kind of morning routine (either a mental, emotional, spiritual, or physical one, or some combination) and stick to it.

Set deadlines and stick to them. When your deadline arrives, if you have not completed that goal, re-evaluate the goal. Figure out why you did not meet it, and set a more attainable goal for next time. The more goals you actually meet, the more you will build willpower and gain new, healthy habits.

You might also want to keep a list of things you have wanted to do for a long time but have not gotten around to, such as house projects or events. If you find yourself with free time (which you will, increasingly!) go to that list, pick one thing, and do it. Keep the list on the refrigerator or somewhere can go to it whenever you are wondering what to do.

The more you are feeling fit, healthy, and whole, the less you will feel like spending time bingeing or vegging. You will start to want to accomplish those goals and have the motivation and energy to do so.

As you begin, try making a list of people who can be your support network. Choose people you can rely on to listen without judgment and reinforce your commitment to better health. If your list seems short, try reaching out to groups in your area and find other like-minded people. In the age of the internet, you can almost always find someone interested in the same things!

You might want to distance yourself from people who do not provide support in your journey. You do not need to shun them or un-friend them, but you can create a healthy space between you by not discussing your goals if you find that they are unsupportive. You can create a list of responses to use in situations when people ask you about your fitness but you do not feel like sharing at the moment. If you know you will receive negative comments about your attempts to change your life, make a small, pleasant comment that does not apologize for your goals or give in to their negativity, then change the subject. You can even try a little self-deprecating humor if you want, but do not make it a criticism of yourself that they can use against you.

The internet is a vast resource of tips and tools for health, wellness, motivation, planners, and other ways to keep yourself on track. Research what works for you and play around. Don't be afraid to try new things and see if they work!

The more you mindfully plan and execute your goals, the better you will feel. Instead of listing ten or twenty things to do every day and then feeling like a failure when you don't finish, keep your day reasonable and then reward yourself when you check everything off your list. As always, schedule time to take care of yourself first and plan the other parts of your life around it.

Best of luck on your journey to fit, fun, and fierce – have fun and enjoy the journey!

Now that you understand the workings of your Mind, Body, and Spirit and their importance in your life, how do you bring them together to increase to become Fit & Fabulous and experience a fit, fun, and fierce life of vitality?

Let's apply what we've learned and make it a new habit. For the next 21 days...

1. **Mind:** Apply your new perspective to your daily living. Be the person you desire to become. No excuses – just do it.

2. **Body:** Workout 3 to 4 times per week to keep your energy active and your body fit. In addition a great way to increase your energy is stimulate your solar plexus with a Yoga charging exercise.

3. **Spirit:** Connect to your inner being to draw upon strength and peace during your transformation.

CHAPTER 6

SUGAR IS CRIPPLING YOU

ow that we have explored the mind, body, and spirit aspects of vitality, let's wrap up by thinking of our wellness on a higher level.

Mindfulness in all these areas of your life will assist you in creating a happier, healthier life in every possible way. Be open to the possibility that more things will change – not just your waistline! Although change can be hard, it is inevitable. We might as well make it a good change.

You have learned to delve your mental, physical, and spiritual traits to improve your overall wellness. The last two chapters of this book are "bonus" chapters to help you come up with your own diet and fitness plans. First, however, let us combine everything we have learned so far into a single whole.

Although this book has discussed a variety of foods, I want to spend a little more time on sugar. Sugar is a good example of what I have illustrated throughout this book because it works on the mental, physical, and spiritual levels.

You can apply what I say here about sugar to other examples, but sugar deserves some extra attention here in the conclusion. Although we typically think of food as merely a physical phenomenon, sugar gets special treatment in this book for the special treatment it gets in our society.

The Standard American Diet includes more sugar than most of us realize. Even our meats, cheeses, and other savory foods are filled with sugar in some form or another. Almost all of this sugar is either highly processed or fully artificial, with high fructose corn syrup being one of the most common ingredients in almost all foods we find on grocery store shelves.

Sugar, then, is a sneaky ingredient that causes much more harm than we realize.

Sugar and inflammation are directly linked, and most diseases are linked to inflammation. That is, less sugar equals less disease.

Further, sugar is directly linked to mental health, as well. Sugar is addictive because it causes us to release dopamine, the "feel good molecule." Digesting sugar also requires you to secrete hormones, which can leave you depleted and imbalanced, especially if you are experiencing hormonal shifts for any other reason, such as menopause. That is why artificial sweeteners are especially bad for you – they require your body to secrete hormones even though there is no sugar to digest.

If your hormones are already struggling due to menopause or even the regular hormonal fluctuations that are common to womanhood, further taxing your hormonal glands with artificial sweeteners is doing you no favors.

Sugar, of course, is known to be bad for us, but we do not always shun it like we should. More pertinently, sugar spikes your energy levels and then drops them again, leaving you craving—you guessed it—more sugar.

The vicious cycle continues, as sugar leaves us stressed, hungry, and ill. Sometimes an unexplained headache or dizziness is really just our body's reaction to sugar (or lack thereof) if you cannot identify another cause. Eating a snack high in protein and fat can help counterbalance it, especially if we pair it with a tall glass of water.

On the subject of water, many of us drink our calories far too often. A sports drink or smoothie is of course highly beneficial if used correctly, but when we drink soft drinks, alcohol, processed fruit juices, and other sugary beverages on a daily basis, we are merely flooding our system with even more sugar.

Further, liquid forms of sugar do not provide fiber or proteins to balance out the sugar in them. Fiber and other food ingredients make sugar more palatable to the body by making it easier to digest, which is why most fruit is healthier than most other forms of sugar.

Drinking your sugar in syrupy soft drinks on a regular basis is dangerous in large quantities. As an occasional treat might be suitable for you (unless you have other health conditions), but soft drinks on a daily basis actually dehydrates you more and puts you at risk for sugar-related health issues.

Sugar is so common that it's no wonder that it is both emotionally and chemically addicting. Not only does it taste incredibly good (as I am sure you well know), it is also one of the first comfort foods people turn to when we are sad.

First, it is a quick carb that provides immediate energy to the body, giving us a pick-me-up that quickly drops us when it wears off a short while later.

Second, one of the first foods you were given as a baby was probably filled with sugar. Fruit, a common baby food ingredient, is filled with sugar, and babies quickly learn to love the sweet taste. Until you were old enough to handle meat and vegetables, you were likely given sugary carbs and sweets, and you were probably also given these things to help you calm down when you were upset.

Again, these parenting techniques are not bad in and of themselves, as anyone who has raised a child knows that you can only do your best and sometimes you need to comfort a baby with food. However, more recent studies in baby-led food weaning advise changing the way we feed infants, for exactly the reasons we are talking about. Teaching a small child to expect a sweet treat when they are sad can be used as a substitute for true emotional support, which can be harmful to their ability to self-soothe.

Like most of us, you probably find yourself reaching for sugar whenever you are upset or craving something tasty. That is because we have learned to associate feeling calm with eating something sweet, and we learned it at a very young age. By itself, this is not a problem. The problem comes in when we allow ourselves to self-soothe with sugar every single time.

In previous eras, it might not have been quite so dangerous to give babies sugar or to eat is as treat, as food overall was less processed, more substantial, and overall less sugary, since white sugar was expensive and rare and typically saved for special occasions. Eating baked goods as a deliberate choice was safer back then because it was something they did as a holiday treat or only once a day, and the rest of their food was relatively sugar free (especially in its highly processed form, white sugar).

By contrast, white sugar today is plentiful and common. It can be found in almost everything we eat, unless it has been replaced with artificial sweeteners like high fructose corn syrup, which are cheaper to produce and can be used in smaller quantities for a much more powerful sweetness punch.

Learning the complex and serious ways that sugar affects our mind, body, and spirit will hopefully help you to limit (or eliminate) your sugar intake on a more permanent basis.

Firstly, the high levels of sugar intake we see today is a recent phenomenon, one we are still adjusting to as a species. For most of human history, sugar was rare and expensive. Ancient cultures used natural sweeteners like honey or dates, but white sugar was not widely available until recently.

Until the 20th century, white sugar was still fairly rare, so most people got by with brown sugar, maple syrup, honey, or other more natural, safer sweeteners, unless it was a special occasion like a holiday or if they were very rich.

In this century, however, sugar is everywhere. If you pick up any random food package, chances are good that it will have multiple chemical sweeteners in it, even if it's a main course (and not a dessert at all). Finding a non-sweetened food (with even no artificial sweeteners added) is virtually impossible, although it can be a fun exercise if you are feeling bored in the grocery store.

To make things even more complicated, sugar now has so many names that you might not even recognize what you are eating as sugary.

Sometimes the label lists it as "sugar," but will also list dextrose or sucralose or any number of "-ose" words. These are also forms of sugar, but will not be listed as the "sugar" on the label. That is why it is crucial to understand the different forms of sugar and their names – so you can recognize them on labels.

Sucrose (or table sugar) is a combination of glucose and fructose. Fructose, the sugar found in fruit, is a natural fruit sugar that most bodies can handle in reasonable amounts, if used as part of a healthy diet. However, our ancestors tended to fruit as a wintertime food, mostly because it was easy to preserve and because it helped them gain extra weight to keep them through the winter months. Fructose is stored in the liver as fat, and under normal circumstances, this is fine.

However, humans no longer live under normal circumstances.

High fructose corn syrup is a sweetener that contains, you guessed it, more fructose than normal. That's because it's a cheap, easy way to get a whole lot of sweetness out of a small amount of product.

It's everywhere. If you have ever tried to avoid high fructose corn syrup, you know that it is not easy to do.

However, high fructose corn syrup is not the only sneaky sugar in our food. Dextrose, a common preservative, is also in many foods that you might expect to be sugar free, such as meat products and other savory dishes.

There are over fifty names for sugar on our food labels, and each one is a different form. Learning to recognize these forms of sweeteners will be important so you can be more mindful of your sugar intake, beyond simply avoiding sugary treats. That way, when you do indulge in your favorite dessert, you can be confident that it's truly the only sugar you have had that day, giving you more freedom to enjoy it.

As mentioned previously, fat has been made the villain in our society. Low-fat, high sugar foods benefit only the companies that produce them and are responsible for a variety of problems in the Western world today. Because low-fat food tastes bland and un-fulfilling, mass-manufacturing companies pump foods full of sugar, instead. The high sugar content makes up for the low-fat content and is much cheaper for them to produce. Meanwhile, sugar has very little nutritional value compared to fat and also can do a great deal of harm in large quantities.

Ironically, the cheaper a food is, the more reliant it is on artificial sweeteners, which cost less than high-quality ingredients. In previous eras, only the upper class could afford sugar on a daily basis. Now, almost everyone eats sugar in almost every meal, whether or not it's a sweet treat.

As you can see, sugar is not only dangerous, it's plentiful, and you are probably eating much more sugar than you think. If you have struggled to maintain a diet in the past, but you were not paying attention to the chemical properties of sugar in your food, you likely struggled because the sugar hijacked you mentally and physically. Freeing yourself of its power will enable you to follow your own dieting choices with ease and joy.

"Breaking up" with sugar will be a freeing experience on a variety of levels. Avoiding sugar in your regular foods will make treats taste sweeter and be more rewarding to you when you do choose to eat them on occasion, and it will let you break your dependency on sugar so you can make more mindful choices about your food and your health.

To live a healthier, happier life in every possible way, look to your sugar intake. Doing your own research about the various types of sugar out there and how to be smarter with your sugar intake is a big step, so do not let yourself get overwhelmed. Sugar is addicting, and it's dangerous, but it is, in our culture, somewhat inevitable.

Some sugars are better for you than others, but this will vary from person to person and is somewhat dependent on what is available in your area. Working with a nutritionist and doing research on the types of sugar that suit your needs is crucial to making sustainable changes that will work for you and your lifestyle.

Becoming a competent reader of labels (even if just the main ideas on it) will assist you in improving your health in so many ways. The crucial skill of understanding food labels will help you in many areas of your life. Learning the names of important food ingredients and teaching them to others is a valuable contribution you can make to your own life and the lives of your family members.

As you do so, you can feel more empowered in your own ability to make your own food choices and eat better whenever and however possible.

Still, do not fret if label reading feels overwhelming or if you are now worrying about how you will ever make any of the changes in this book. If you do nothing else for your overall wellness, being aware of and decreasing your sugar intake will be an enormous gift you can give yourself and your family members.

Cutting down on sugar as much as possible will make a significant difference in your life. Sugar is chemically and mentally addicting, and it is also significantly unhealthy. The rising levels of sugar intake in America today are tied to our growing obesity and illness rates.

The good news is that as you do the mental and emotional healing work discussed throughout this book, your sugar cravings will lessen over time. You likely find it hard to avoid sugar by sheer force of will right now, and that is okay. As you begin to recognize the underlying mental and emotional processes that lead you to turn to sugar, which you now know is both physically and mentally addicting, you will need to turn to sugar less and less.

Instead, you can enjoy a variety of healthy foods with the occasional sugary treat thrown in. Your body will adapt to your newer, stronger lifestyle and start to crave food that nourishes you, instead of food that depletes you. Your overall wellness will increase in a body that looks good and feels good, sometimes even without any reason at all.

As you begin replacing the sugar in your life with other, more wholesome foods, you can begin to make the other changes outlined in this book.

Further, as you make the changes necessary to heal on the mental, physical, and spiritual levels, you will find yourself healthier and happier overall and will not need to self-soothe with sugar quite so much.

The next time you are craving something sweet, ask yourself: am I really hungry? Or am I upset? Choosing to take a relaxing bath or calming walk instead might do the trick, especially if you pair it with a protein-packed wholesome snack. Giving your mind, body, and spirit the nourishment it needs will train it to expect true support whenever you are feeling badly, instead of the quick pick-me-up of sugar that ultimately leaves you crashing down again. A sustainable happiness is one that lasts beyond the pint of ice cream or the quart of cookie dough. True vitality means feeling good consistently, not just when it's easy.

Throughout this book, I have described the mental, physical, and spiritual aspects of healing that will lead you to a healthier, happier you. You can be fit, fun, and fierce at any age by following the techniques found in this book.

The most important thing to remember is that you are already fabulous. Do not let anyone tell you otherwise. So take what you've learned, stir up your energy and go out and intent to have more fun in your life. Intent to try something new often!

One last thing, if you've enjoyed this book please leave a review on Amazon and keep in touch...

MayaMFitness

Maya_M.Fitness

CHAPTER 7

BONUS#1

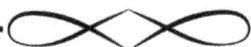

AT HOME WORKOUT PLAN

Monday's Workout	Sets	Reps
Bodyweight Squat	3	10
Rear Bodyweight Lunge	3	10
Single Leg Resistance Band Deadlift	3	6
Push Up	3	6-10
Resistance Band Lat Pull Down	3	10
Dumbbell Row	3	10
Plank	3	30 Secs

Wednesday's Workout	Sets	Reps
Resistance Band Deadlift	3	10
Dumbbell Goblet Squat	3	10
Glute Bridge	3	12
Donkey Kicks	3	12
Resistance Band Row	3	10
Resistance Band Shoulder Press	3	8-10
Ab Crunch	3	15

Friday's Workout	Sets	Reps
Push Ups	3	6-10
Resistance Band Lateral Raise	3	10
Resistance Band Pull Down	3	10
Resistance Band Row	3	10
Bodyweight Squat	3	10
Glute Bridge	3	15
Side Planks	3	30 Secs Each

GYM WORKOUT PLAN

Train on Monday, Tuesday, Wednesday, Thursday

Monday: *Back/ Biceps* **Do 4 sets of 12-15 repetitions each.**

Tuesday: *Chest/ Triceps* **Do 4 sets of 12-15 repetitions each.**

Wednesday: *Shoulders* **Do 4 sets of 12-15 repetitions each.**

Thursday: *Legs/ Glutes* **Do 4 sets of 12-15 repetitions each.**

All 4 days: Abs

Choose two or three abs exercises each day and do 3 sets of 25–30 repetitions each.

Monday, Tuesday, and Wednesday: Cardio

Each day do 30 minutes of high-intensity intervals (including a five-minute warm up and cool down) on a stair machine or walk briskly on a treadmill set to a 50% incline. Do one minute at 80–90% maximum heart rate (8–9 on a scale of 1–10), followed by one minute of slower-paced active rest.

GYM EXERCISE PLAN

For accountability and fitness plans with progressions check out

www.mayamfitness/coaching

Abs	**Legs**
Weighted Crunch	Stationary Lunge
Hanging Knee Raise	Hack Squat
Kneeling Cable Crunch	Seated Hamstring Curl
Vertical-bench Leg Raise	Lying Hamstring Curl
Back	**Shoulders**
Close Grip Pull down	Lateral Raise
Seated Cable Row	Front Plate Raise
Bent Over Dumbbell	Shoulder Press
Biceps	**Triceps**
Barbell Curl	Rope Pull downs
Dumbbell Hammer Curl	Triceps Kickbacks
Cable Preacher Curl	Cable Overhead
Chest	
Barbell Bench Press	
Flat-bench Dumbbell Press	
Cable Crossover	

CHAPTER 8

BONUS #2

∞

12 WEEK WEIGHT LOSS MEAL PLAN

Weeks 1-4

Follow the meal plan outlined here, which also includes Food Swaps. In addition, try to consume at least one gallon (16 cups) of water a day. A limited amount of sodium helps regulate body fluids, so don't be afraid to use low-calorie condiments like mustard and hot sauce.

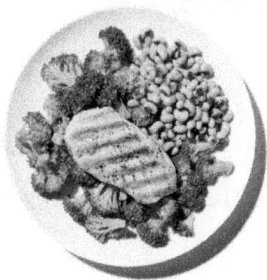

Breakfast

- » 4 egg whites
- » ⅓ cup (uncooked) instant oatmeal
- » 10 almonds

Totals: 240 calories, 20g protein, 22g carbs, 8g fat

Mid-Morning Snack

- » 4 oz skinless, boneless chicken breast
- » 3 oz sweet potato, boiled or baked, without skin
- » ½ oz English walnuts, shelled

Totals: 258 calories, 26g protein, 17g carbs, 11g fat

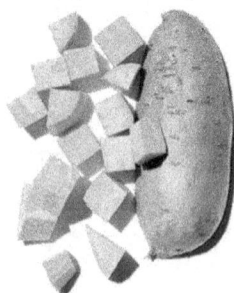

Lunch

- » 4 oz skinless, boneless chicken breast
- » ½ cup long-grain brown rice
- » 1 cup chopped broccoli, boiled or steamed

Totals: 263 calories, 29g protein, 34g carbs, 3g fat

Midday Smoothie

- » 1 scoop whey protein isolate
- » 1 cup almond or skim milk & ice
- » Honey to taste
- » ½ large (8») banana
- » 1 tbsp natural peanut butter

Totals: 271 calories, 29g protein, 19g carbs, 9g fat

Dinner

- » 5 oz cod
- » 1 white corn tortilla
- » 1 cup sliced zucchini, boiled

Salad:

- » 2 cups mixed greens
- » 10 almonds, crushed
- » ¼ cup cherry tomatoes, quartered
- » ¼ cup red onion
- » 2 tbsp. balsamic vinegar

Totals: 328 calories, 32g protein, 32g carbs, 9g fat

Evening Smoothie

- » 1½ scoops whey protein isolate
- » 2 cups water & ice

Totals: 158 calories, 38g protein, 0g carbs, 1g fat

Daily totals: 1,518 calories, 174g protein, 124g carbs, 40g fat

Food Swaps

Freshen up your daily diet by switching out the foods in the plan with some of the choices below. Remember to keep portion sizes consistent so your nutrient intake and calorie count stay on track during each phase.

	Food	Portion	Calories	Protein	Carbs	Fat
POULTRY*	Chicken (boneless, skinless)	4 oz	100	23g	0	2g
	Turkey (boneless, skinless)	4 oz	120	28g	0	1g
FISH*	Tilapia	4 oz	108	23g	0	2g
	Pollock	4 oz	104	22g	0	1g
	Haddock	4 oz	98	21g	0	1g
	Cod	4 oz	93	20g	0	1g
	Sole/Flounder	4 oz	103	21g	0	1g
CARBS†	Brown rice	½ cup	108	3g	2g	1g
	Sweet potato	4 oz	86	2g	20g	0
	Yam	4 oz	132	2g	31g	0
VEGGIES	Asparagus	1 cup	40	4g	7g	0
	Broccoli	1 cup	55	4g	11g	1g
	Spinach	1 cup	41	5g	7g	1g
	Brussels sprouts	1 cup	56	4g	11g	1g
	Green beans (uncooked)	1 cup	31	2g	7g	0

*Measured uncooked. †Measured cooked, unless otherwise stated.

Weeks 5–8

In this phase, you'll trim calories slightly to help drop body fat, although protein intake will stay steady to make sure your metabolism remains high and you're not losing muscle tissue along with the fat. Feel free to keep referring to the Food Swaps list as desired. Keep up your fluid intake, drinking at least one gallon of water per day.

Breakfast

- » 3 egg whites
- » 2 oz 99% fat-free ground turkey breast
- » ⅓ cup (uncooked) instant oatmeal

Totals: 214 calories, 29g protein, 19g carbs, 3g fat

Mid-morning Snack

- » 4 oz skinless, boneless chicken breast
- » ⅓ cup long-grain brown rice

Totals: 172 calories, 25g protein, 15g carbs, 2g fat

Lunch

- » 4 oz skinless, boneless chicken breast
- » 1 cup black-eyed peas, boiled
- » 1 cup kale or spinach

Totals: 355 calories, 40g protein, 47g carbs, 3g fat

Midday Snack

- » 4 oz 99% fat-free ground turkey breast
- » 2 white corn tortillas
- » 1 oz avocado

Totals: 257 calories, 31g protein, 20g carbs, 6g fat

Dinner

- » 4 oz cod
- » 1½ oz avocado

Salad:

- » ½ tbsp. extra-virgin olive oil
- » 2 tbsp. balsamic vinegar
- » 2 cups mixed greens
- » ¼ cup tomato
- » ¼ cup onion

Totals: 290 calories, 23g protein, 17g carbs, 14g fat

Evening Smoothie

- » 1 scoop whey protein isolate
- » 1 cup water & ice
- » 1 tbsp. organic flaxseeds

Totals: 160 calories, 27g protein, 3g carbs, 5g fat

Daily totals: 1,448 calories, 175g protein, 121g carbs, 33g fat

Week 9-12

Your carbohydrate and protein intake drop a bit more during this phase, reducing your total calories and helping your body dig further into its fat stores. (Healthy fat intake stays steady, though, to help you feel full and to fuel your muscles.) Keep drinking plenty of water so you stay well hydrated. And don't forget to swap out for your favorite foods!

Breakfast

- » 5 egg whites
- » ⅓ cup (uncooked) instant oatmeal

Totals: 188 calories, 22g protein, 20g carbs, 2g fat

Mid-morning Snack

- » 4 oz skinless, boneless chicken breast
- » 1 cup raw green beans
- » 10 almonds

Totals: 200 calories, 27g protein, 10g carbs, 8g fat

Lunch

- » 4 oz skinless, boneless chicken breast
- » ⅓ cup long-grain brown rice

Salad:

- » 2 cups mixed greens
- » ¼ cup tomato
- » ¼ cup onion
- » 1 tbsp. balsamic vinegar

Totals: 227 calories, 26g protein, 26g carbs, 2g fat

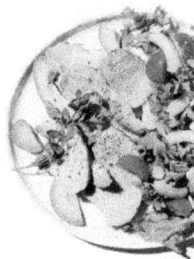

Midday Snack

- » 4 oz skinless, boneless chicken breast
- » 3 oz sweet potato, boiled or baked, without skin
- » ½ oz English walnuts, shelled

Totals: 258 calories, 26g protein, 17g carbs, 11g fat

Dinner

- » 4 oz skinless, boneless turkey breast
- » 1 oz avocado
- » 10 almonds

Salad:

- » 2 cups mixed greens
- » ¼ cup cherry tomatoes, quartered
- » ¼ cup yellow onion
- » 2 tbsp. balsamic vinegar

BEST AND WORST FOODS FOR WEIGHT LOSS

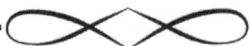

BEST FOODS

GRAPEFRUIT

Grapefruit is a great snack. It is high in water content, so it's useful for hydration and has a healthy quantity of vitamin C, which is required for skin health, to keep that glow all summer. What's more, studies show grapefruit may help promote weightloss by reducing insulin levels and boosting your metabolism.

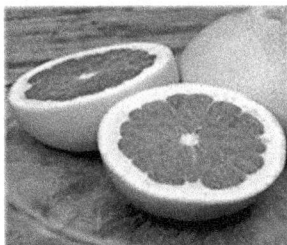

LEAFY GREENS

"Not only are leafy greens a great way to add volume to your meals without the calories, but they are chock full of nutrients (vitamins A, C, K, folate, calcium, iron, magnesium, potassium, and fiber) and easy to incorporate into your day," says Mary Dinehart-Perry, a registered dietitian and clinical trials director for Zone Labs, Inc. She recommends swapping out iceberg for spinach in your salads, adding mustard greens or collards to your

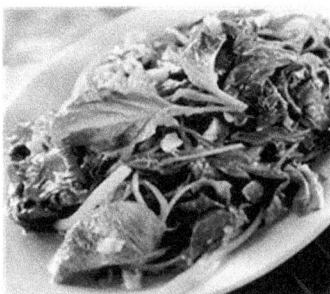

soups, or dishing up a side of sautéed kale to fill up, fight disease, and look fab in your bikini.

RED BELL PEPPERS

"This beautifully colored vegetable is bursting with antioxidants (especially vitamin C and beta-carotene) to help your body fight off infections," says Margaux J. Rathbun, a certified nutritional therapy practitioner and creator of nutrition website Authentic Self Wellness. "They are also stimulating for the digestive system and have been shown to be metabolism-boosters, helping you to lose unwanted pounds. They are perfect for dieters when eaten raw or prepared in a juice concoction."

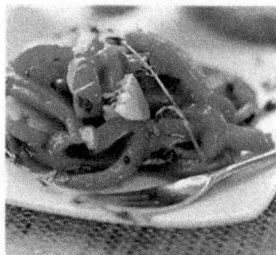

GREEK YOGURT

Just one 6-ounce container of plain Greek yogurt has 0g fat and 18g protein, plus it contains probiotics and supplies 20 percent of your calcium needs, Dinehart-Perry says. Unlike other yogurt brands (which can be packed with sugar), Greek yogurt works for gluten-free, vegetarian, or diabetic dietary needs, and even those with lactose intolerance may be able tolerate yogurt better than milk. Can't handle it plain? Add some fresh fruit or turn it into a healthy parfait.

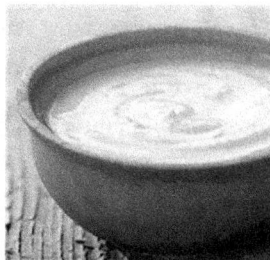

QUINOA

Looking for a healthier alternative to rice or pasta? Try Quinoa! "Quinoa is actually a seed, but the texture is very much like a grain," says Lauren Kelly, staff nutritionist for The Bar Method in Montclair, New Jersey. "Unlike grains, this super food is a complete protein (it contains all nine essential amino acids), loaded with fiber, vitamins, minerals, and antioxidants."

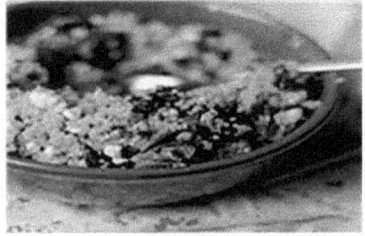

SALMON

"Salmon is naturally low in calories, saturated fat, and sodium and a good source of protein; what really makes it stand out is its omega-3 fatty acid content," Dinehart-Perry says. "Omega-3 fatty acids, especially EPA and DHA, are becoming increasingly popular for their anti-inflammatory benefits."

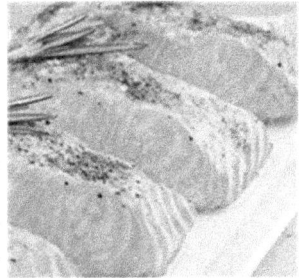

RAW NUTS

"Raw nuts are high in healthy fats, vitamins, minerals, and antioxidants," Kelly says. "Eating raw nuts (like almonds, walnuts, and Brazil nuts) regularly has shown to reduce your risk of heart disease and possibly prevent breast cancer." Kelly recommends steering clear of roasted and

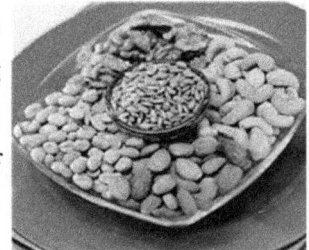

salted nuts and sticking with raw varieties for the best slimming (and health) benefits.

STEEL CUT OATS

Steel cut oats are the least processed type of oatmeal and are packed with fiber, protein, and whole grains, Kelly says. "Oats have shown to help reduce cholesterol and help maintain healthy blood sugar levels." Prepare plain, steel cut oats and add honey and/or fresh fruit for a little sweetness.

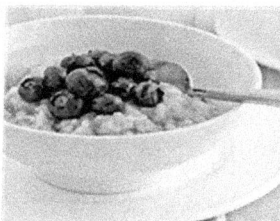

PEPPERMINT

"Peppermint works to reduce bloating and indigestion and soothe the GI tract all around," says Rachel Berman, registered dietitian and director of nutrition for CalorieCount.com. Try mixing up some iced peppermint tea or add a few mint leaves to your water.

FRIED EGGS

Eggs are chock full of amino acids and the combo of protein and fat helps you feel full and avoid overeating. "The protein in the egg helps to build muscle and burn fat which tones your physique," says Ilyse Schapiro, a registered dietitian and owner of a private nutrition practice specializing in weight loss in New York City. And you don't have to save them

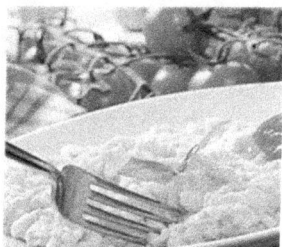

for breakfast. Eggs are incredibly versatile and can be added to almost any meal or snack. Try any (or all) of these 20 quick and easy ways to cook eggs.

BLACKBERRIES AND STRAWBERRIES

Berries are packed with antioxidants and fiber, so they'll keep you feeling full on fewer calories, Shapiro says. Plus, the antioxidants will help you with your workouts by improving blood flow to your muscles. Sounds like a great summer snack to us! Or when you>re on the go, drop by Jamba Juice for an Orange Berry Antioxidant juice.

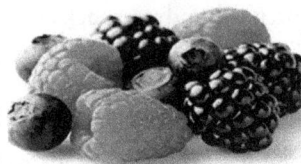

CHEWABLE CELERY

Still hungry after a meal? Chew on celery sticks! They'll help decrease fluid retention and fill you up without adding many calories to your daily total, Berman says.

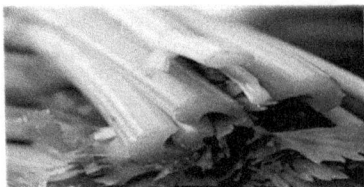

FRESH PINEAPPLE

This tropical, naturally sweet fruit is perfect for summer, and it's great for your bikini bod too. "Pineapple contains bromelain, a digestive enzyme that can help reduce gas," Berman says.

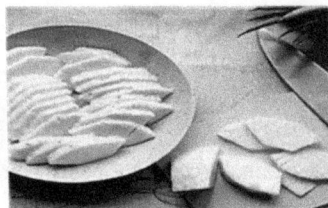

BRUSSELS SPROUTS

A nutritious, low-cal veggie, Brussels sprouts may not be the most bikini-friendly, Berman says. "While they contain fiber and nutrients, they can also cause gas and GI expansion, so incorporate them slowly into your diet to reap high fiber benefits." They will help you stay healthy and bikini body ready, just don't eat them right before you head to the beach for the best bikini belly.

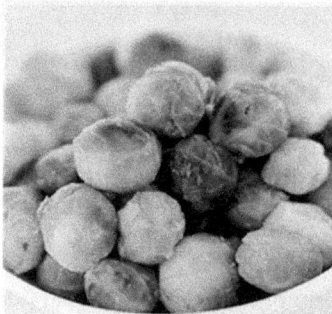

WORST FOODS

SUSHI

Sushi may seem like a good, low-cal meal option, but not all sushi is created equal. "When it comes to ordering sushi this summer, stay with simple rolls," Rathbun says. Steer clear of deep fried rolls and those covered in sauce and choose slimmer sashimi and veggie rolls with brown rice instead.

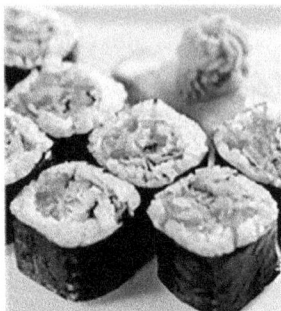

PRETZELS

Even though they're low fat, Berman says this is a empty calorie snack you can skip. "Pretzels are high in sodium, which can result in water retention and bloating. Not to mention, pretzels are devoid of any wholesome nutrients and therefore will leave you hungry and wanting more."

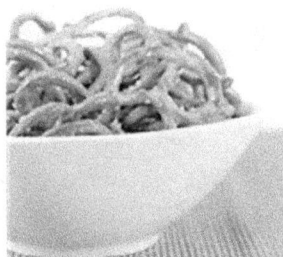

STORE BOUGHT SMOOTHIES

Don't be fooled by a healthy reputation. Sipping on a store bought smoothie may not be any better for your waistline than a fully loaded sandwich!

"Many people don't know that commercial smoothies can have 600 to 1000 calories a pop," Shapiro says. "Not only is that more calories than a typical meal, but the sugar content can be through the roof, which your body stores as fat." You're better off grabbing some real fruit instead, or if you love a good smoothie, make your own at home so you can control what goes in the blender.

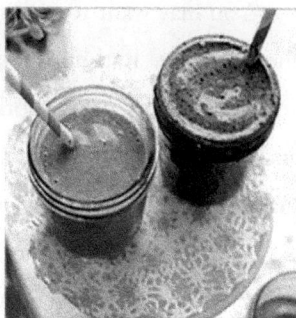

MARGARINE

Switching from butter to margarine isn't going to be any better for your bikini body. "This once popular spread was thought to help us maintain a healthy weight, but it turns out margarine contains trans fat (the "bad fat") which contributes to not only weight gain but cardiovascular disease," Rathbun says. Stick with lower-cal toppings like Greek yogurt and all-fruit spreads instead of margarine and butter whenever possible.

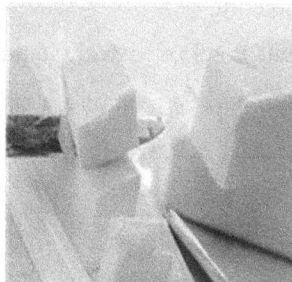

FRUIT JUICES

You may want to rethink that glass of OJ in the morning, Rathbun says. "Most fruit juices contain a lot of sugar (both naturally occurring and some that companies add) that can cause a massive spike in our blood sugar levels. Fruit juice is also loaded with calories, something we want to pay attention to when maintaining a healthy weight.»

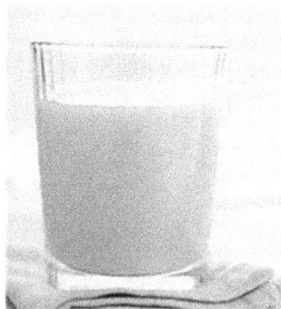

If you just can't do without juice, Rathbun recommends diluting it with some water to help slash the calorie and sugar content.

SOY SAUCE

Avoid belly bloat and water retention by steering clear of soy sauce, Rathbun says. Soy sauce is loaded with sodium that will cause our bodies to retain water." Try using a high-quality sesame oil dressing or liquid amino acids to add flavor.

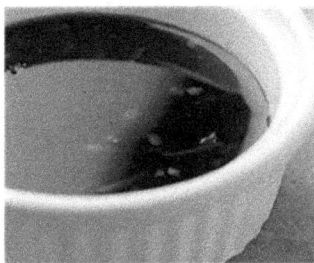

WHITE FLOUR PASTA

"Eating any product made out of white flour causes your blood sugar to spike and then crash—the body recognizes white flour as sugar and stores it completely," Shapiro says. "Because of its effect on your blood sugar, when you crash, you crave more

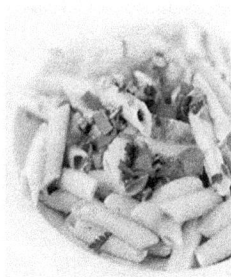

food, specifically in the form of sugar, a total blow to your waistline. There are so many delicious whole wheat breads and pastas on the market, there is no need to waste calories on this dead end food."

BACON

Forget what low-carb diets tell you. Kelly says bacon is one of the unhealthiest processed meats out there, thanks to its high sodium and nitrate contents.

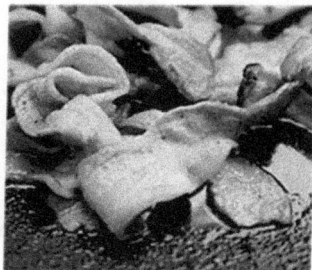

"Nitrates are preservatives that are used in processed foods to maintain their color. When these nitrates are baked or fried at high temperatures, they become carcinogenic."

Yikes! If you really love bacon, look for leaner, low-sodium options that are nitrate free, and enjoy it in an equally decadent recipe that won't ruin your diet).

PIZZA

Okay, so it's not that surprising, but we're all guilty of giving in to the convenience of frozen pizza for dinner. Try to limit those indulgences to the cold seasons. "Frozen pizzas are loaded with sodium and preservatives; most are made with

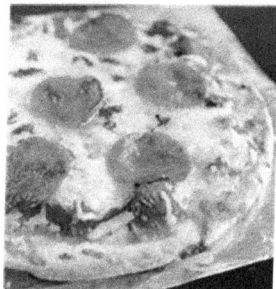

white flour that has been bleached and reacts in your body just like sugar, which can lead to weight gain.

The good news is you don't have to give up pizza altogether: make your own with whole-wheat pizza dough, reduced-fat cheese, and tons of veggies.

ICE CREAM

Again, not so shocking, but ice cream is synonymous with summer! It can also rack up your daily totals by supplying up to 300 calories, one third of your daily recommended fat intake, half your saturated fat, and one third of your daily cholesterol intake, Dinehart-Perry says. And that's just in one half-cup serving (and who eats only a half cup?). Dinehart-Perry recommends trying non-fat or low-fat varieties instead or switching to sorbet, sherbet, or bars made with 100-percent fruit or Greek yogurt.

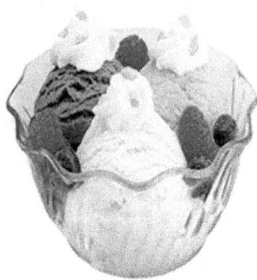

CONCLUSION

$$\infty$$

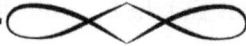

Tips To Beginning Your Transformation Today

I n closing, I'll cover a few extra tips and tricks that will help tremendously in transforming your body. Some tips might require you to adjust your lifestyle entirely. However, they are of great assistance in losing weight.

Exercise

It's the surest and most natural way to lose weight. Exercising can be done in so many ways to fit into your daily activities. For instance, you can decide to cycle to and from your workplace or shopping center instead of taking a bus. On the other hand, you can opt to use the stairs instead of the elevator. Other activities like walking, jogging, and running will also contribute to weight loss.

You can also make exercising fun, like playing basketball with your peers or kids, going on long walks with your loved ones and many more fun activities that eventually will burn calories. On the other hand, you can structure an exercising routine every day that will involve at least 30 minutes of cardiovascular exercises.

Remember, exercises on top of burning up fat and calories also help in building a lean muscles mass which is essential for the body's metabolic rate.

Consume the right drinks

If it's not possible to quit alcohol entirely, limit yourself to a maximum of two on isolated cases when you have to take alcohol. Alcohol has no nutritional value to the body and the body usually uses it as its first energy source. Eventually, the food consumed ends up being stored as fat in the body. Alcohol also influences you to eat the wrong type of foods, usually junk foods that are high in calories. It's therefore essential to avoid alcohol consumption, or to limit its consumption, as much as possible.

Similarly, avoid fruit drinks and soda. Instead, opt for sugarless drinks and plenty of water. Water suppresses the regular urges to eat and consequently help you lose some weight. It also keeps the body hydrated, which is ideal for nutrients' release to the body.

Green tea is also favorite beverage for people on a weight loss program. Studies have demonstrated that consuming green tea leads to more calories being burnt faster than those who do not consume it.

Consume the right foods

Eat the right foods that will not contribute to weight gain but rather to weight loss. Grapefruit has been found effective in helping people lose weight. Consuming half a grapefruit three times a day burns more calories by boosting the body's metabolism. On the other hand, avoid or minimize on the consumption of fats, especially animal fats as they are high in cholesterol. Opt for skim milk and low-fat cheese. Similarly, consume lean meat, preferably white meat. In addition, opt for unprocessed foods as their calories and fat content is lower. On the other hand, if you have to consume processed food, like bread, opt for the whole grain bread as its high in dietary fiber content. Fiber assists in burning calories.

Also, things to avoid are, refined sugar containing products and junk food. Look for sugar substitutes to use in the place of sugar. Junk food is low in nutritional value and high in calories content. Avoid it as well. However, ensure you consume plenty of fruits and vegetables and minimize on starch products for an almost ideal body weight.

For a full book of great receipts please check out my Vegetarian Lifestyle Recipe book: DOMINATE: Optimize your body for vitality and longevity in 21 days.

D epending on your current activity level and time commitment, choose to be active and exercise 3 to 6 days per week. Highlight your days (Monday, Tuesday, Wednesday, etc...) of choice and set aside a specific uninterrupted time to complete your workout. Use the above workout plan or create one of your own.

Place a checkmark in the box below after completion.

TRACK YOUR CONSISTENCY

Month # 1

Date	Sun.	Mon.	Tues.	Wed.	Thurs	Fri.	Sat.
1							
2							
3							
4							

Month # 2

Date	Sun.	Mon.	Tues.	Wed.	Thurs	Fri.	Sat.
1							
2							
3							
4							

Month # 3

Date	Sun.	Mon.	Tues.	Wed.	Thurs	Fri.	Sat.
1							
2							
3							
4							

References

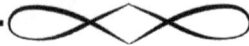

Introduction:

[1] Stevenson, B. & Wolfers, J. (2009). The paradox of declining female happiness. *American Economic Journal, 1*(2), 190-255.

[2] Killbourne, J. (2010). *Killing us softly: Advertising's image of women.* Retrieved from: https://shop.mediaed.org/killing-us-softly-4-p47.aspx

[3] "Ernestine Shepherd" (2020). Retrieved from https://ernestineshepherd.net

[4] Levine, P. A. (2010). *In an unspoken voice: How the body releases trauma and restores goodness.* Berkeley: North Atlantic Books.

Chapter 1:

[5] Srivastava, S. (2003). Personality is not set by 30; It can change throughout life, say researchers. *American Psychological Association.* Retrieved from

[6] Helmstetter, S. (2014). *The power of neuroplasticity.* Scotts Valley: CreateSpace Publishing.

Chapter 2:

[7] House, J. M. (2008). *Peak vitality: Raising the threshold of abundance in our material, spiritual and emotional lives.* Santa Rosa: Elite Books.

[8] Nagpal, R., Mainali, R., Ahmadi, S., Wang, S., Singh, R., Kavanagh, K., Kitzman, D. W., Kushugulova, A., Marotta, F., &Yadav, H. (2018). Gut microbiome and aging: Physiological and mechanistic insights. *Nutrition and Healthy Aging, 4*(4), 267-285.

[9] Sonnenburg, J. & Sonnenburg, E. (2016). *The good gut: Taking control of your weight, your mood, and your long-term health.* New York: Penguin Books.

[10] Sheikh, K. (2017). How gut bacteria tell their hosts what to eat. *The Scientific American.*

[11] Sonnenburg, J. & Sonnenburg, E. (2016). *The good gut: Taking control of your weight, your mood, and your long-term health.* New York: Penguin Books.

[12] Gershon, M. D. (1998). *The second brain: A groundbreaking new understanding of the nervous disorders of the stomach and intestine.* New York: Harper Collins.

[13] Morell, S. F. (2017). *Nourishing fats: Why we need animal fats for health and happiness.* New York: Hachette Book Group.

[14] Baumeister, R. F. & Tierney, J. (2011). *Willpower: Rediscovering the greatest human strength.* London: Penguin Books.

[15] He, Y., Yin, J., Lei, J., Liu, F., Zheng, H., Wang, S., Wu, S., Sheng, H., McGovern, E., & Zhou, H. (2019). Fasting challenges human gut microbiome resilience and reduces Fusobacterium. *Medicine in Microecology, 1*(2), 1-5.

[16] Paoli, A., Mancin, L., Bianco, A., Thomas, E., Mota, J. F., & Piccini, F. (2019). Ketogenic diet and microbiota: Friends or enemies? *Genes, 10*(7), 534.

[17] Taubes, G. (2016). *The case against sugar.* New York: Knopf Doubleday Publishing Group.

[18] Morell, S. F. (2017). *Nourishing fats: Why we need animal fats for health and happiness.* New York: Hachette Book Group.

[19] Mayer, E. (2018). *The mind-gut connection.* New York: Harper Collins.

[20] Bush, B. & Hudson, T. (2010). The role of cortisol in sleep. *Natural Medicine Journal, 2*(6).

[21] McKeown, P. (2015). *The oxygen advantage: The simple, scientifically proven breathing techniques for a healthier, slimmer, faster, and fitter you.* New York: Harper Collins Publishing.

Chapter 3:

[22] Benabou, R. & Tirole, J. (2003). Intrinsic and extrinsic motivation. *Review of Economic Studies, 40,* 489-520.

Chapter 4:

[23] American Cancer Society. (2015). Water fluoridation and cancer risk.

[24] Arlene Semeco: The 19 Best Prebiotic Foods You Should Eat. June 8, 2016.

[25] Lakowski, E. R. (2018). What are the risks of sitting too much? *Mayo Clinic.*

[26] www.womenfitnessmag.com/the-best-workouts-for-women-over-40/

Chapter 5:

[27] Dyer, W. (2020). *Dr. Wayne Dyer*.

Chapter 6:

[28] Taubes, G. (2016). *The case against sugar*. New York: Knopf Doubleday Publishing Group.

[29] Reeves, S. (2008). Baby-led weaning. *Nutrition Bulletin, 33*, 108-110.

[30] Harvard Health. (2011). Abundance of fructose not good for the liver, heart.